Healing
is
Voltage

Healing Eye Diseases

Healing
is
Voltage

Healing Eye Diseases

Jerry Tennant, MD, MD(H), MD(P)

Contents

Chapter	Title	Page #
1	Who is Dr. Tennant	1
2	Healing is Voltage	8
3	Tennant BioModulator®	89
4	Dental Toxins	111
5	Bowling Ball Syndrome	133
6	Nitric Oxide	150
7	Humic/Fulvic Acids	159
8	Healing Eye Diseases	173
9	Cataracts	191
10	Macular Degeneration	199
11	Glaucoma	215
12	Uveitis	241
13	Summary	248

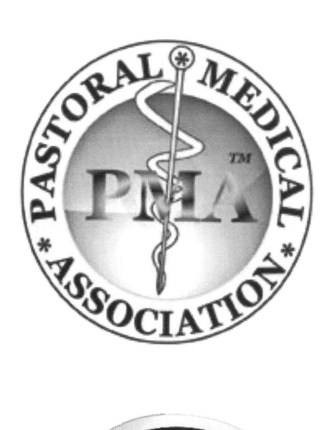

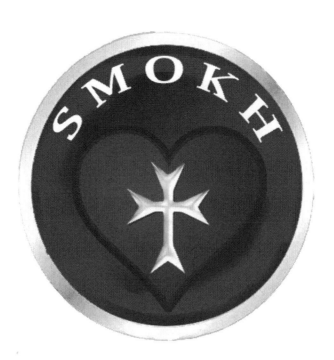

Introduction

book implies that you release Jerry Tennant and related parties from any liability, real or imagined, from any adverse events suffered by the reader.

About This Book

This book is a part of the **Healing is Voltage** series. It follows the book <u>Healing is Voltage, The Handbook.</u> In that book, I discussed the things I learned about how the body really works and what it takes to make it well.

I have practiced ophthalmology since 1965. I was trained in the usual allopathic paradigm. It teaches doctors to focus primarily on the organ of interest and to refer patients to other doctors interested in other organs if they seem to have a problem. I remember that years ago a local internist was furious at me because I was looking at cholesterol and blood pressure to see if they were causing macular degeneration. He insisted that as an ophthalmologist, I had no business looking at cholesterol levels, ECG's, or blood pressure. Medicare first told me I could look at the circulation in the carotid arteries because they supply blood to the eye. Later they fined me because they said I was the only ophthalmologist trying to be sure that the eye got enough circulation to be healthy. It continues to amaze me that modern medicine is so specialized that everyone forgets that the various parts of the body are connected and influence each other. That is part of why the best doctors I could find didn't know how to get me well when I was too sick to work.

The advantage for me as an ophthalmologist in trying to figure out better ways to treat eye diseases was that learning how the body really works has taught me a different paradigm. Looking at eye disease from this new paradigm makes things obvious to me that I would never have figured out with the limitations of only using medications and surgery to correct diseases.

Because the way to cure eye diseases is the same as the way to cure other diseases of the body, I have copied and reproduced several chapters from Healing is Voltage, The Handbook for the benefit of those that have not read that book. If you have read that book, you may wish to skip directly to the chapters in this book about eye diseases.

As you read this book, remember that we get well primarily by making new cells, not by correcting those that aren't working. Making new cells requires adequate voltage (-50 millivolts), the raw materials necessary to make new cells, correction of cellular software, and removing the toxins that damage old and new cells.

FOREWORD

My introduction to the concept of electro-magnetic measurements in biological systems came while I was studying for my M.D. at Yale University School of Medicine. In order to graduate from this particular medical school, one must write a thesis. I chose, in 1959, Dr. Harold Saxton Burr, Professor of Neuro-anatomy, as my advisor for my thesis project. Dr. Burr, at that time, was acknowledged as a lead investigator and proponent of The Electro-magnetic Field Theory in Biology. During my studies with Dr. Burr, I was exposed to the concept of taking electronic measurements with a direct current potentiometer on various living organisms, including humans, to measure electrical changes that accompanied changes in those biological systems.

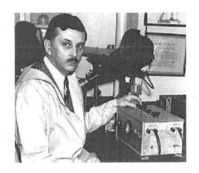

Subsequently, I became familiar with the knowledge that creating an electrical field, such as that reported by Dr. Robert O. Becker and Dr. Andrew Bassett, an orthopedic surgeon at Columbia University School of Medicine, could be of assistance for healing processes in the clinical condition of non-union of orthopedic fractures. Therefore, I understood that electronics in living systems could not only be measured but, indeed, these systems could be modified by an electrical field.

With the information provided above as a background, I was, perhaps, more receptive than most physicians would be to accept the idea that electronic stimulation could be of benefit in certain clinical conditions. My first hand exposure to the benefit of electronic stimulus as therapy was a very rapid recovery from a previous knee injury after being treated with a Russian electronic device, called a SCENAR, utilized by Dr. Jerald Tennant, in January 2003.

I had met Dr. Tennant in the late 1970's and arranged, with assistance of Dr. John Corboy, for him to present the first intraocular lens course with hands on guidance ever taught in Honolulu, Hawaii. Our friendship had been established at that time and, therefore, I was interested in the Energetic Medicine workshop he was presenting at the Hawaii Meeting on Maui in 2003. My inquiry about the course at the Faculty dinner led to his treating me for the injury which I had acquired while indulging in my favorite sport of surfing. The dramatic improvement in my knee function led me to purchase the Russian device and take Dr. Tennant's course taught in Dallas, Texas that year.

I do not presume to understand or profess all the concepts that are presented in this book authored by Dr. Tennant. The SCENAR, and the other electronic devices, subsequently designed by Dr. Tennant, such as the Tennant BioModulator®, are classified by the FDA as class 2 accepted devices for the relief of pain and inflammation. Over the past eight years, I have, in my ophthalmic practice personally treated with these devices over 275 patients who had painful ocular syndromes with approximately 85% success. The syndromes have included pain after corneal injury, iritis, migraine, and postoperative discomfort after strabismus and cataract surgery. The pain syndrome, known as post-herpetic neuralgia (pain after shingles), has been especially responsive. In some patients, the pain in the skin had plagued the patient for over 10 years. You can imagine the gratitude of these patients when there is a complete relief, after treatment by an electronic device, for a condition that has not responded to drugs and other modalities of treatment. I thank Dr. Tennant for introducing me to this new paradigm of medical treatment. We may not understand the mechanisms of healing at this point, but, in the final analysis, **results trump theory in any case**.

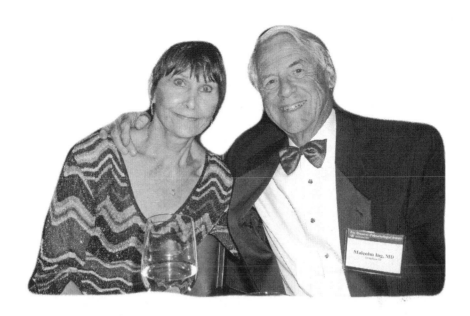

Malcolm R. Ing, MD

Clinical Professor of Surgery

Division of Ophthalmology, Department of Surgery

John A. Burns School of Medicine, University of Hawaii

1 Who is Jerry Tennant?

I graduated as valedictorian of high school at age 16. I completed my junior and senior years simultaneously by taking home study courses. I completed college except for three hours in 2 1/2 years at Texas Tech University. I received the Phi Kappa Phi Award and the premed of the year award. I attended the University of Houston School of Optometry before medical school. I was accepted into Southwestern medical school at age 19. I graduated in the top 10 at age 23.

I completed a residency in ophthalmology at Harvard Medical School/Massachusetts Eye and Ear Infirmary and the Southwestern Medical School/Parkland Hospital system between 1965 and 1968.

I am board certified in ophthalmology and ophthalmic plastic surgery.

I was the director of ophthalmic plastic surgery clinic at Parkland Hospital.

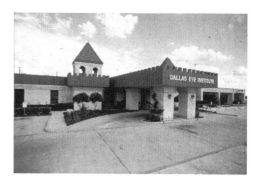

I was the founder/ director Dallas Eye Institute.

I have a Doctor of Natural Medicine license from the Pastoral Medical Association (MD(P)). I am licensed in Arizona by the Board Of Homeopathic And Alternative Medicine MD(H)).

I hold patents for medical devices including intraocular lenses, surgical instruments, etc.

I was co-founder of the Outpatient Ophthalmic Surgical Society, and I taught most of the ophthalmologists how to do outpatient eye surgery in the 1980s.

I was one of the first surgeons in United States to place intraocular lenses in eyes after cataract surgery. I taught those techniques around the world.

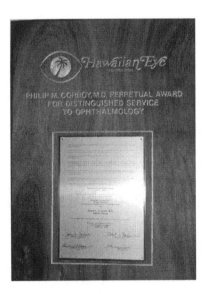

I am one of the few in the world to receive the Corboy Award for Advancements in Ophthalmology.

I received the American Academy of Ophthalmology Award for my contributions to ophthalmology.

I've written several books about cataract surgery and lifestyle management.

The Order of Saint Sylvester is intended to award Roman Catholic laymen who are actively involved in the life of the church, particularly as it is exemplified in the exercise of their professional duties and mastership of the different arts. It is also conferred on non-Catholics, but more rarely than the Order of St. Gregory.

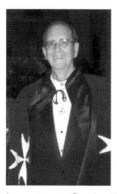 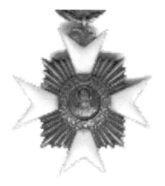 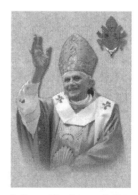

I am not Catholic. However, I was awarded the Order of St. Sylvester by Pope Benedict XVI in July 2008 for my contributions to medicine.

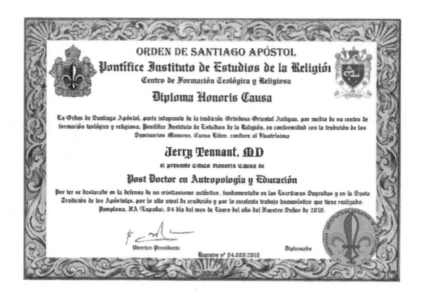

I received a PhD (hon) in Anthropology and Education from the ORDEN DE SANTIAGO APÓSTOL, an ancient religious Order of Spain, under the priory of Monseñor Basilius Adao Pereira, Priorato Real de los Caballeros de

Jerusalem, Pontífice Instituto de Estudios de la Religión under The Order of Santiago, more properly the Military Order of Saint James of the Sword.

I currently work at the Tennant Institute for Pastoral Medicine, an Ecclesiastical Private Expressive Association, as defined by law, and provide service as a Pastoral Health Practitioner and Counselor.

See www.tennantinstitute.com

I practiced ophthalmology from 1964 to 1995. I did much of the FDA study for the VISX excimer laser. I performed about 1000 cases in the United States and about 2000 cases abroad from 1991 to 1995.

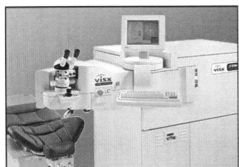 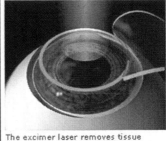

The excimer laser removes tissue from the cornea's internal layers.

http://www.ohsuhealth.com/cei/images/lasik_laser.jpg

I did the majority of the study for the FDA to get approval for the VISX laser used in LASIK surgery. I performed about 1000 cases in the US and about 3000 cases abroad.

What we didn't know at the time was that the laser would not

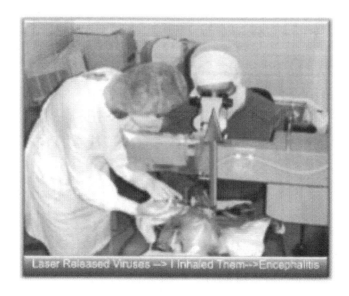

Laser Released Viruses --> I Inhaled Them-->Encephalitis

kill viruses. The laser would strike the cornea, release viruses, and they would float upward through my mask into my nose and into my brain. I developed encephalitis, neuropathies, a low platelet count, and other nervous system defects in 1994. I could see a patient to know what was wrong with them, but I couldn't remember how to write a prescription. I also developed spastic movements and that prevented me from safely performing eye surgery. I had to quit work on November 30, 1995.

For almost 7 years, I slept about 16 hours per day. Remember that I had viruses in my brain and viruses in my spleen. Note in the picture that my dog Tigger would sleep on my head, and my dog Pooh would curl up next to my spleen. They seemed to know where my voltage was low, and they were my constant "electron donors"!

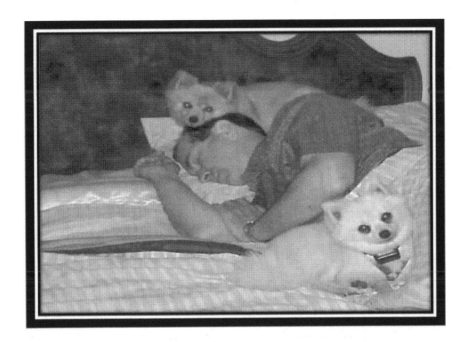

I went to see the best physicians I could find around the country. They simply told me that I had three viruses in my brain and in my spleen and that nothing could be done for me. They told me to go home and do the best I could do. They had nothing to offer.

I had about 2-3 hours per day that I could think clearly enough to understand a newspaper. Then like a light switch, it would turn off and I couldn't understand it any more. During the time I could think, I would try to figure out how to get myself well. It occurred to me that if I could figure out how to make one cell work, I could make them all work. Thus I began reading cellular biology books, something I hadn't done for about 30 years.

The cellular biology books all had a statement or two about the need for cells to run at a pH of 7.35 to 7.45. I didn't know what that really meant, but for some reason that resonated with me.   That started my journey to the understanding that Healing is Voltage! I'll discuss that in the next chapter.

2 Healing is Voltage

You will recall that I began my journey toward getting well by recognizing that cells are designed to run between a pH of 7.35 and 7.45. I also began my journey with the idea that if I could figure out how to make one cell work I could make them all work.

The following chart shows you the requirements for a cell to work properly.

Requirement	Range for Cell	Abnormally High	Abnormally Low
Glucose	80-110 mg./dl	Diabetes	Hypoglycemia
Temperature	98.6-100 F.	Fever	Hypothyroidism
Blood Pressure	120-140/80 -90	Hypertension	Hypotension (dizziness)
pH	7.35-7.45	Throbbing Pain	Chronic Pain
Oxygen	$paO^2 > 95\%$	Doesn't occur	Anaerobic metabolism -- >Lactic Acid -- >Lowered pH

We doctors are trained to pay particular attention to things that are abnormally high. For example, we watch carefully for a high blood sugar (diabetes); however, we rarely think about hypoglycemia unless a patient is dizzy or faint. We watch carefully for high temperature indicating fever, but we are not trained that a low temperature indicates hypothyroidism. We watch carefully for high blood pressure and are insensitive to the fact that low pressures due to over-exuberant prescription of medication is causing our patients to be dizzy. We rarely look at pH levels or oxygen levels unless the patient is in intensive care.

I want to focus on the importance of pH. When I was trying to figure out how to get well, I couldn't remember a lot about pH. I remembered that it was something about acid/base balance but I knew very little more than that. So I began to read about pH. What I discovered is that pH (shorthand for "potential hydrogen") is really a measurement of voltage.

When electrons are running through a conductor like a copper wire, they are there or not. If the switch is on, you have an electron donor. If the switch is off, there are no electrons.

However, a solution provides a different situation. The solution may be an electron donor or an electron stealer. One measures the voltage of the solution with a sophisticated voltmeter. By convention, if the solution is an electron donor, one puts a minus sign in front of the voltage. If, however, the solution is an electron stealer, one puts a + in front of the voltage. For example, if your pH voltmeter measures +150 millivolts, it means that the solution is an electron stealer with 150 millivolts of stealing power. If your pH voltmeter measures -200 millivolts, it means that the solution is an electron donor with 200 millivolts of donating power.

After measuring the voltage of the solution, one can convert that to a logarithmic scale called pH. A voltage of +400 mV is the same as a pH of zero. A voltage of -400 mV is the same as a pH of 14. A solution that is neither an electron donor nor electron stealer is called a pH of seven.

pH	0	7	14
Voltage	+400 mV	0 mV	-400 mV

With this understanding, one can see that a pH of 7.35 is the same as a voltage of -20 mV. A pH of 7.45 is the same as a voltage of -25 mV. Thus we see that all cellular biology texts tell us that cells are designed to run between -20 and -25 millivolts of electron donor status!

The following chart begins to help us understand the difference between electron donors and electron stealers as it relates to the human body.

Electron Stealer	Electron Donor
Causes damage	Can Do Work
pH 0-6.9	pH 7.1 - 14
Acidic	Alkaline
Free Radical	Antioxidant
Positive Pole	Negative Pole

Electron Stealer	Electron Donor
Destructive	Constructive
Spins Left	Spins Right

Electron stealers cause damage, are a pH from 0 to 6.9, are acidic, are free radicals, are the positive pole, are destructive, and at the atomic level spin left.

You will hear statements like "all disease occurs when you are acidic." What this is really saying is that all disease occurs when your voltage is low or in an electronic stealer state.

You will hear statements like "alkalize or die". What this means is that you must have electrons available to do work or your cells will die.

A free radical is a molecule that is missing electrons. It is like a mugger looking for someone's purse to steal. When a free radical steals electrons from the cell, it damages the cell.

An antioxidant is a molecule capable of giving away electrons. Thus, when your mother says "eat your vegetables" she is saying that the vegetables contain electrons that are good for you.

We maintain our health and heal primarily by making new cells. To make a new cell requires a voltage of -50 mV.

Cell Voltage	Cell pH	
-50	7.88	Make New Cells
-45	7.79	
-40	7.7	
-35	7.61	Normal for kids
-30	7.53	
-25	7.44	Normal for adults
-20	7.35	
-15	7.26	Tired
-10	7.18	Sick
-5	7.09	
0	7	Change polarity
+5	6.91	
+10	6.83	
+20	6.65	
+30	6.48	Cancer occurs

Salivary and urinary pH are about 0.8 pH units less than cell pH. Salivary pH is a rough indicator of cellular voltage. Urinary pH is a rough indicator of the voltage in the fluids around cells. When normal, both should be 6.5. If you add 0.8 to 6.5, you get a pH of 7.3. This equates to -20 millivolts.

Now let's consider my thumb. My thumb is running at a voltage of -25 mV. It is pink, feels fine and works well. Now I hit it with a hammer. The thumb is red, swollen, hot, and has a pulsing pain. It has automatically gone to -50 mV. This is necessary to make new cells needed to replace the ones I damaged with a hammer. At -50 mV, blood vessels dilate and dump raw materials such as proteins, carbohydrates, fats, vitamins, minerals, etc. into the neighborhood. I need these raw materials to build new cells. I also need -50 mV to

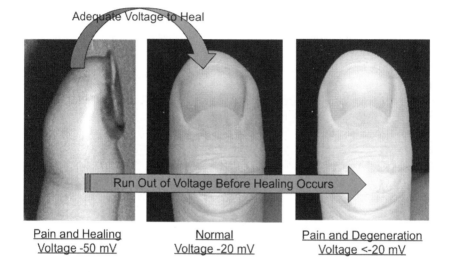

Adequate Voltage to Heal

Run Out of Voltage Before Healing Occurs

Pain and Healing	Normal	Pain and Degeneration
Voltage -50 mV	Voltage -20 mV	Voltage <-20 mV

have the energy to turn these raw materials into new cells.

As soon as I finish making enough cells to replace those I damaged with the hammer, my thumb goes back to -25 mV. It is normal and I am happy.

Now let's assume that I ran out of voltage before I was able to make enough new cells to replace those I injured with a hammer. My voltage dropped to -10 millivolts. Now I am stuck in chronic disease. I cannot heal unless I can make new cells. I cannot make new cells unless I have -50 mV and all the raw materials I need to make new cells. In chronic disease, my thumb hurts all the time, it is white, and doesn't work very well.

Thus we see that chronic disease is always defined by having low voltage. One cannot cure chronic disease without inserting enough electrons to achieve -50 mV. One must also have the raw materials necessary to make new cells and to eliminate the toxins or infections present that will damage the new cells. One can take all of the medications you like and do as much surgery as you like but you will not heal unless you have -50 mV, raw materials, and lack of toxins.

Without the ability to achieve -50 mV and the necessary raw materials to make new cells, you cannot maintain your health and you suffer aging and chronic disease. You also are unable to repair injuries so they can also lead to chronic disease. You don't need drugs to heal. You need to make new cells that work to heal. To make good cells, you need voltage and a good diet. You also need to remove toxins from your body that damage cells and make you obese.

Once one begins to understand that chronic disease and healing are controlled by voltage, one must ask the following questions:

1. How do cells normally get voltage?
2. How do cells store voltage?
3. Why did my voltage drop enough to allow me to get sick?
4. How do I measure the voltage of organs?
5. What do I do when I find the voltage is low?

There are several bad things that happen when voltage drops. The obvious one is that organs simply don't have enough horsepower to do their job. Another is that they don't have the energy to get rid of toxic waste and it begins to accumulate.

Remember that at -50 mV, there is a pulsing pain. When you have low voltage, it simply hurts all the time. Thus pain is simply a symptom of abnormal voltage. You correct it by correcting the voltage.

If you put a tube into a glass of water and began bubbling oxygen into the water, the amount of oxygen that will dissolve in the water is dictated by the voltage of the water. As voltage is raised, more oxygen will dissolve in water. However, as voltage drops, oxygen comes out of solution and leaves the water.

Our cells are 70% water. Thus as voltage begins to drop in ourselves, oxygen leaves the cells. This has serious consequences.

Our cells contain a process for turning fatty acids into glucose. They are processed through a series of chemical reactions called the Krebs cycle. The end result is a rechargeable battery called ATP. As ATP provides electrons to keep the cell functioning, it becomes a discharged, rechargeable battery called ADP.

When oxygen is available, for every unit of fatty acids run through the Krebs cycle, we create 38 molecules of ATP. However, if oxygen is unavailable, only two molecules of

ATP are created for every unit of fatty acids. Thus as voltage drops, and oxygen levels drop, our metabolism goes from "38 miles per gallon to 2 miles per gallon." Thus it is very difficult for cells to have enough energy to function with such inefficient metabolism.

Another problem of decreased oxygen is infections. Our bodies contain perhaps 1 trillion microorganisms. However, most of these are inactive as long as oxygen is present. However, when oxygen levels drop, these bugs wake up. The first thing they want to do is have lunch. And, they want to have you for lunch.

Since these bugs don't have teeth, they must put out digestive enzymes to dissolve you so that they can acquire the nutrients from the cells.

One of the problems has to do with these digestive enzymes. Let's assume that you have a Streptococcus bacteria having lunch on your tonsil. You, of course, recognize this as a sore, painful throat. We all know, however, that the digestive enzymes produced by these Streptococcus bacteria can enter our bloodstream and cause damage to our heart valves. They can also damage your joints. The same process can happen anywhere in the body. Let's assume you have low voltage in your gallbladder. This means that your gallbladder will hurt, have decreased oxygen, and inefficient metabolism, and have bugs having lunch on the gallbladder. The toxins produced by these bugs can enter the bloodstream and cause brain damage. You may have infections in your large intestine, in your sinuses, or other places causing damage an autoimmune problem.

However, it is simply bugs having lunch because your voltage and thus your oxygen levels are low.

I have seen a number of patients with a diagnosis of lupus. A blood test called the ANA test is used to make the diagnosis of lupus. If you correct the voltages in such patients, their symptoms go away and their ANA test goes back to normal.

As voltage continues to drop, it will go from an electron donor to electron stealer status. This is known as a change in polarity. When voltage drops to +30 mV, you have cancer.

It is generally taught in Western medicine that the blood is sterile. This is because placing blood into a Petri dish does not normally show growth. Generally speaking, only bacteria that have cell membranes reproduce in Petri dishes. However, if you look at blood under a high-powered microscope without the blood stains or other chemicals you will easily identify many microorganisms. These microorganisms do not have cell membranes. As voltage and oxygen levels drop, and as toxins build up in the system, you will see these organisms change from spherical to rod-shaped to yeast like and finally fungus with hyphae. The association of finding fungal like forms in the blood with the development of tumors was reported as long ago as 1840 and has continued to be reported ever since. Although the existence of these forms has generally been denied by most microbiologists and oncologists, the development of the German microscope known as the Ergonom makes these denials no longer credible. This microscope is capable of 15,000 to 40,000 power and allows one to see even viruses

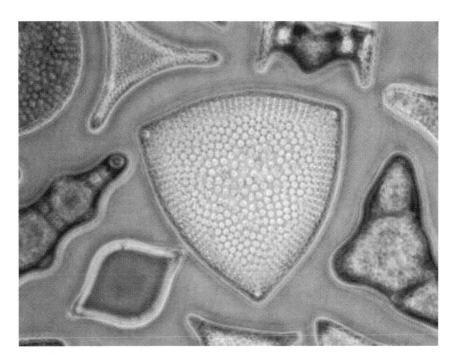

in their live state. Please look at the videos at
www.grayfieldoptical.com

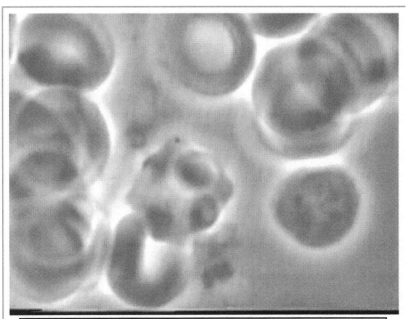

L-forms in red blood cells   Phase Contrast Microscope

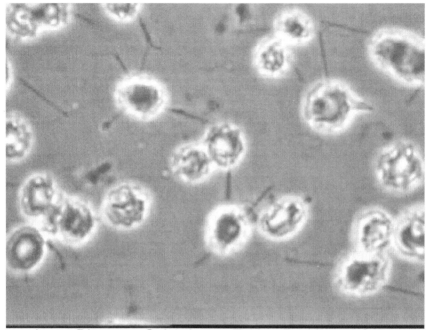

Lyme Disease: Spirochetes Exiting Red Blood Cells
Phase Contrast Microscope

HOW DO CELLS NORMALLY GET VOLTAGE?

There are many ways that the body is intended to get electrons. However, our modern culture has tended to eliminate most of these sources.

The Earth is a large electromagnet. If you take the electrodes of a voltmeter and stick them into the dirt, you will measure voltage. An area of high voltage always causes electrons to flow to an area of low voltage. If your body has lower voltage than the earth, walking barefoot on the dirt or grass will cause electrons to flow from the earth into your body, recharging you. However, if you walk with shoes, this cannot occur.

Ion	Volts	Millivolts
Fluoride	2.85	2,850
Peroxide	1.77	1,770
Chloride	1.36	1,360
Ferric	0.76	760
Copper +	0.52	520
Copper++	0.34	340
Hydrogen	0	0
Chromium	-0.41	-410
Ferrous	-0.44	-440
Zinc	-0.76	-760
Aluminum	2.23	2,230
Magnesium	-2.71	-2,710
Sodium	-2.87	-2,870
Calcium	-2.89	-2,890
Barium	-2.92	-2,920
Potassium	-2.99	-2,990
Cesium	-3.02	-3,020
Lithium	-3.04	-3,040

Water from the ground contains electrons. We call this "alkaline water." However, when place chlorine and fluoride into the water it turns it into an electron stealer. Thus every time we drink such water, it steals electrons from us. The water we should be drinking should contain electrons and be clean and free from toxins. Again, you can test your water to see if it is electron donor or electron stealer by simply placing the electrodes of the voltmeter into the water. If the voltmeter shows minus voltage, the water is an electron donor. If the voltmeter shows plus voltage, the water is an electron stealer.

If you stick a voltmeter into a raw potato, you will measure voltage. However, if you bake a potato or freeze the potato and then insert the voltmeter, most of the voltage will be gone. Unprocessed food contains voltage. Once we process food, most of the voltage disappears. We are designed to eat unprocessed food so that it brings its own electrons with it. When you eat food that has been processed, your body must provide electrons from other sources to digest it. You can actually tell the quality of food such as vegetables by simply using a voltmeter to compare the voltage in one product versus another.

Remember that voltage always moves from an area of higher voltage to an area of lower voltage. When my wife and I hug each other, there is obviously an emotional element. However, there is also an issue of pure physics. The one of us with the lower voltage will get a donation of electrons from the other one. As we continue to hug, soon we will be the same voltage.

This process continues when any two living things touch. For example, if I hold a dog or cat and I am lower voltage than the dog or cat, the animal will donate electrons to me. Then it will run outside, recharge itself, and bring me some more voltage. If I lean against a tree, the tree will donate voltage to me.

Moving water is always an electron donor. Still water is an electron stealer. Thus taking a shower will energize me whereas taking a bath will make me tired. Swimming in the ocean will give you electrons, but swimming in a chlorinated pool will steal voltage from you.

Moving air is an electron stealer. Thus people often feel tired if they sleep under a fan. Riding in a convertible is great fun, but you are always tired when you get to your destination.

If you take a voltmeter that measures in millivolts and hold it in the air inside your home, you will measure a small amount of voltage. Now take it outside. You will find there is much more voltage out in the sun.

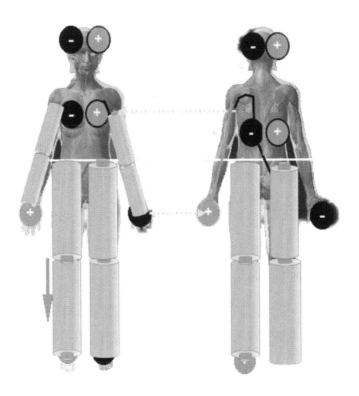

If you take a quartz crystal and squeeze it with a pair of pliers, it will emit electrons. This is called the piezoelectric effect. Our muscles are piezoelectric crystals. Thus when we exercise, our muscles create electrons. The muscles are also rechargeable batteries. Thus the movement of our muscles re-charges our muscle batteries. Exercise is a major way the body acquires electrons.

There is a pump within the skull and down the spine called

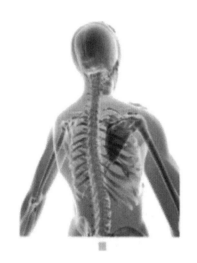

the craniosacral pump. Each time this pump activates, it sends a surge of electrons through the body.

Thus you can see that the human is designed to get voltage primarily the way our grandparents got it. They worked out in the sun, drank water from a well, ate unprocessed foods, weren't afraid to touch the earth with their hands or feet, hugged their family, leaned against a tree or stood in moving water while they were fishing, and weren't afraid to stand in the rain.

Common Ways Electrons are Taken From the Human Body

1. Acidic water (tap water, chlorinated water, fluoride, most bottled water)

2. Carbonated beverages
3. Caffeinated beverages (pop, coffee, tea)
4. Alcoholic beverages
5. Cooked food
6. Processed food
7. Healers/doctors who touch their patients lose electrons to patient
8. Hugs: transfer electrons from one person to another
9. Parent holding sick child: child gets well quicker and parent left tired
10. Moving air: wind, air conditioning, fans, convertibles, and hair dryers

How Do Cells Store Electrons?

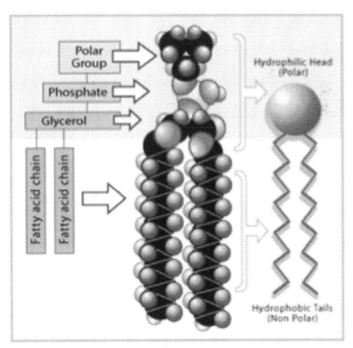

Cell membranes are made up of opposing layers of fats called phospholipids. This unusual fat is made up of a ball with two legs. The ball is an electron conductor. The legs

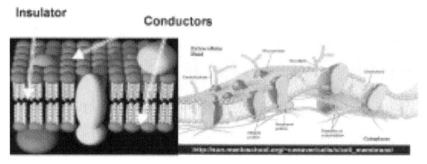

Cell Membrane is a Capacitor = "Battery Pack" for Cell

Cell Membrane With Opposing Molecules of Phospholipids

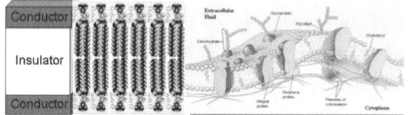

Two Conductors Separated by an Insulator Creates a Capacitor

are insulators.

Anytime two conductors are separated by an insulator, you have an electronic device called a capacitor. Capacitors are designed to store electrons. Thus cell membranes serve as "battery packs" for the cells.

Liquid Crystals

Dr. Bruce Lipton has recently discovered that the cell membrane also serves as a liquid crystal. The molecules in solid things stay in one location. An example of a solid is a crystal. However, in liquids, the molecules move about. In some substances called liquid crystals, the molecules can move about but act like solids. This means that liquid crystals are neither a solid nor a liquid. Thus the name seems strange in that we are calling a solid a liquid when we

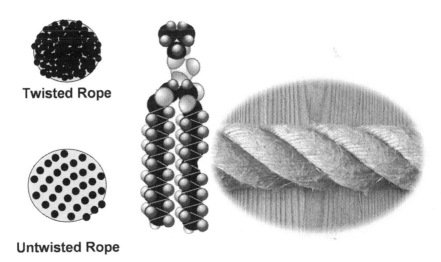

Twisted Rope

Untwisted Rope

say, "liquid crystal". We are basically saying, "Liquid Solid".

Liquid crystals are influenced by electric current and/or temperature. Certain liquid crystals have elements that are twisted. When one applies electricity to these liquid crystals, they begin to unwind. One can use this characteristic to use them to either block the passage of light through them or allow the light to pass This depends upon whether the elements are twisted or untwisted.

The thing that determines whether the elements are twisted or untwisted can be anything from a magnetic field to a surface that has grooves in it. An LCD is made with two plates of polarized glass, one in front and one in back. The back one is polarized 90 degrees from the front one. In between these two plates are filters coated with liquid crystals. The orientation of the crystals is aligned with or opposed to the passage of light depending upon the voltage applied. It is like having a rope with its fibers twisted tightly so light cannot pass down its length or a rope with its fibers untwisted so that there are spaces between the fibers that allow light to pass down its length. The function is very much like a rotating diaphragm that opens or closes depending upon whether voltage is present or not.

One can see that the phospholipids that make up a cell membrane have legs that can twist or untwist to permit light or water or other molecules to be blocked or pass through the cell membrane. They open and close depending upon the voltage applied.

Semiconductors

Carbon, silicon and germanium are elements that are called semiconductors. Each has four electrons in their outer shell. This allows each atom to attach the four other atoms in a nice crystalline structure called a lattice. The carbon lattice is called a diamond.

Carbon, silicon, and germanium in their crystal state are electronic insulators. Because they do not have free electrons (all are bonded to each other), they insulate rather than conduct electricity. However one can turn these insulators into what are called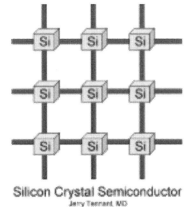

Silicon Crystal Semiconductor
Jerry Tennant, MD

"semiconductors" by adding impurities to the crystals. This process is called "doping".

As you can see in the graphic of a portion of the periodic table, carbon, silicon, and germanium are in a column. In the column next to them are nitrogen, phosphorous, and arsenic. To the left, the column contains boron, aluminum, and gallium.

Arsenic and phosphorous each has five outer shell electrons. When you place one of them into a lattice of carbon, silicon, or germanium (each of them has four electrons), there is an extra electron per set of four atoms. This extra electron can move from place to place turning the insulating crystal into a "semiconductor" that allows some

IIIA	IVA	VA
5	6	7
B	C	N
13	14	15
Al	Si	P
31	32	33
Ga	Ge	As

electric current to flow through it. Since this semiconductor has a negative charge, it is called an "N-type". If you add boron or gallium to a crystal of carbon, silicon, or

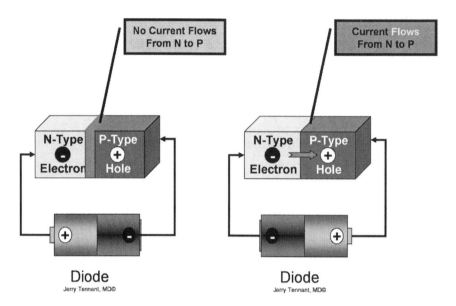

Diode

Jerry Tennant, MD©

Diode

Jerry Tennant, MD©

germanium, you have a different kind of semiconductor.

Since boron and gallium each have only three electrons in the outer shell, binding them to carbon, silicon, or gallium (each has four electrons) creates a hole in the latticework. This hole is searching for electrons and accepts electrons that wander by. This creates a positive charged semiconductor called a P-type semiconductor.

Diodes

When you place a negative and a positive semiconductor against each other, you have what is called a diode. What is unique about a diode is that it allows electric current to flow in one direction but not the other. It is a one-way street for electric current whereas conductors like copper allow the electric current to flow either direction.

When you put a voltage source like a battery as you see in the left part of the graphic, the plus part of the battery attracts and hold the electrons from the negative N-type semiconductor and the minus pole of the battery attracts and holds the holes in the positive P-type semiconductor. The result is that no current flows through the semiconductors. Devices that allow current to flow in one direction but not in the other direction are called diodes.

If you change the battery to the configuration you see in the right side of the graphic, electrons flow from the battery into the N-type semiconductor and then into the holes of the P-type semiconductor with the net effect that current is flowing through the diode.

Transistors

If you use three elements instead of two, you have a transistor. You can use two N-type with a P-type in the middle or two P-type with an N-type in the middle. The most commonly used type is two N-type and one P-type as it is easiest to use this format in a silicon sheet to make a chip. A transistor normally blocks the flow of electricity though it, acting as a switch. However, when you apply voltage to the center layer, a large amount of voltage can move though the transistor making it act as an amplifier. A small current can turn a larger current on and off.

As you can see, the phospholipids of the cell membrane act like a transistor and a microprocessor. A piece of silicon that can hold thousands of transistors is called a silicon chip.

**N-P-N Transistor Can Function
As a Switch or Amplifier**

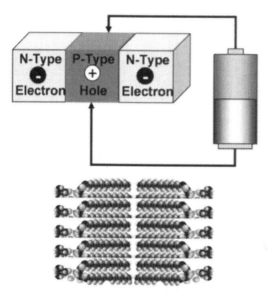

**Phospholipids of Cell Membrane
Form N-P-N Transistors → Microprocessor Chip**

With transistors acting as switches, you can create Boolean gates, and with Boolean gates you can create microprocessor chips.

For an excellent discussion of LCD's and Transistors, see:
http://www.howstuffworks.com/lcd1.htm

The Peripheral Cytoskeleton and Tesla's Resonating Circuits

In 1895, Nikola Tesla invented the Tuned Circuit or Resonating Circuit. It is a capacitor and a coil wired in parallel. Wired in parallel means that the components are on a square as you see in the diagram. Capacitors (abbreviated as "C") store electrons. Coils provide inductance (abbreviated as "L". This is known as an "LC" circuit.

Parallel Tuned Circuits are used in radio and other electronics to couple Resonant Energy from one circuit to another in transmitters and receivers. This is the system used by the cell membrane and peripheral cytoskeleton to couple energy from to

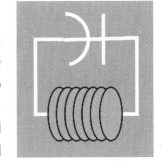

cell and into the cell. As you will recall, the cell membrane is made of two opposing layers of fat molecules that create a capacitor. Just under the cell membrane is a maze of protein called the peripheral cytoskeleton. These two are wired together in parallel in what is known as an RC circuit =

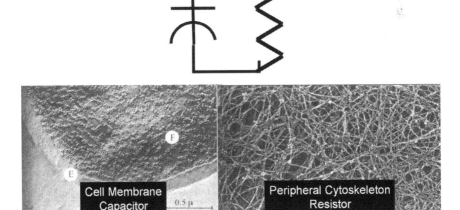

Cell Membrane Capacitor   0.5 µ   Peripheral Cytoskeleton Resistor

resistor/capacitor circuit.

RC circuits work much like your checking account and savings account. In the photo, assume cash is coming into the top of the circuit, the resistor is your checkbook and the capacitor is your savings account. As the cash comes in, it flows through your checking account to pay your bills. Any cash left over is transferred into your savings account. On months in which there isn't enough cash coming in to pay your bills, you take some out of savings and transfer it into your checking account to keep things going. So it is with an RC circuit. Electrons come into the circuit and flow through the resistor (peripheral cytoskeleton of the cell) to keep energy flowing into the cell so it can do its work.

When there are more electrons being delivered by the perineural system, the acupuncture system, water, ionic transfer, etc. than are needed to supply the requirements of the cell, the excess is stored in the capacitor (cell membrane). When the cell is inflamed, delivery of more electrons is reduced because the cell becomes somewhat isolated from the delivery systems by the edema. Thus the cell must operate on the electrons stored in the cell membrane. This is the same as "running on battery power".

Thus you see that the control of voltage into the cell is controlled by a Tesla RC circuit.

A series tuned circuit is used to electrically "stretch" or "shorten" an antenna or waveguide transmission line so that the length of the antenna or waveguide will match the length of the incoming wave. For example, radio stations each put out a different frequency or wavelength. If you have a wire that is exactly the same length, the energy from the radio signal will be absorbed and you will hear that station on your radio. Thus to hear all the radio stations in your area, you would need a separate wire for each station to match the wire lengths and wavelengths. However, if you attach your wire to the series coil above and make the capacitor variable in power, it changes the effective length of the wire. That is the tuning knob on your radio. In the body, extracellular fluid (impedance) and organs (capacitance) are wired in series as a series tuned circuit.

We now see that the cell membrane is the BRAIN of the cell. It is a CAPACITOR that stores voltage for the cell to use. It is a MICROPROCESSOR that controls the functions of the cell by interacting with the environment around the cell. It is a LIQUID CRYSTAL that can open and close to allow things to enter the cell or keep them out and also allow things to exit the cell or keep them in. It is part of a TESLA RESONATING CIRCUIT that allows it to communicate with other cells.

Remember that every cell is designed to run at about a negative 20-25 millivolts. When cells need to repair themselves, the voltage is increased to 50 millivolts. This is controlled by the cell membrane/peripheral cytoskeleton resonating circuit. Since the electrons necessary to allow this to happen are stored in the fat of the cell membrane, the fat is critical to the cell being able to do its work at -20 mV and to repair itself at -50 mV. Without an adequate amount of good fat, the cell membranes can't function and thus the cell can't function. You must also remember that cells replace themselves frequently. If you don't give the cell new building materials including adequate amounts of good fat, the cells will have to make new cells with materials from the worn-out cell it is replacing. Building new things using worn-out parts creates a new thing that doesn't work much better than the old one it is replacing.

As you can see, cell membranes must be made with good phospholipids (fats) for them to work. Making them with plastic fats prevents this from working correctly. Since all of the brain and nervous system, the liver and every cell membrane are made of fat, you must eat lots of good fat to keep making good cells. A normal person is about 20-25% fat. That means you need to eat about 20-25% of your normal body weight in fat every eight months because your body completely replaces itself every eight months.

Trans Fats ("Plastic Fats")

In the 1920's food merchants were concerned about the amount of money that was lost due to spoilage. They wanted to find ways to keep food from spoiling. They found that if they put certain chemicals like nitrates into the food, it was less likely to spoil. The problem is these chemicals preserve cells in your body as well as the food so they stop working. Cells that don't work are what we call disease.

Next, food manufacturers found that if they cook fats at about 350 degrees for about five hours, it turns the fats into something that is similar to plastic. The fats that are processed in this way are called "partially hydrogenated fats" or "Trans Fats" or "Plastic Fats". If you will look in your pantry, you will find that about 40% of what is there contains partially hydrogenated fats. When you eat these plastic fats, your cell membranes become made of plastic. Cell membranes made of plastic won't hold voltage. Without voltage, your cells can't work.

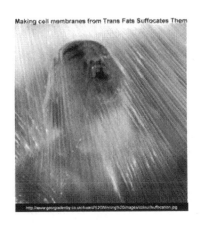
Making cell membranes from Trans Fats Suffocates Them

Think of a cell with a plastic membrane. It is like wrapping the cell in cellophane. The cell sends out signals that it is hungry. The body sends glucose and insulin to the cell. However, they can't get through the plastic membrane. The cell continues to signal that it is hungry and the body continues to send insulin and glucose. Soon the cell is surrounded by insulin and glucose, but the cell is still hungry. This is known as insulin resistance and Type II diabetes. The cell membrane becomes so saturated with glucose that it begins to off-load it into fat cells. Thus people who continue to eat plastic fats get fatter and fatter.

Guess what happens to a brain made of plastic? It doesn't work well and we have depression, chronic fatigue, attention-deficient, brain fog, etc. Guess what happens to a liver that is made of plastic? It can't clean toxins out of your system and the toxins build up causing things like fibromyalgia. Without a functional liver, your immune system fails and you get all sorts of chronic infections.

Another type of toxic Fat is Canola Oil. Here is a summary of a few facts regarding Canola Oil:
   1. It is genetically engineered rapeseed.

2. Rapeseed is lubricating oil used by small industry. It has never been meant for human consumption.
3. It is derived from the mustard family and is considered a toxic and poisonous weed, which when processed, becomes rancid very quickly.
4. It has been shown to cause lung cancer.
5. It is very inexpensive to grow and harvest. Insects won't eat it.
6. Some typical and possible side effects include loss of vision, disruption of the central nervous system, respiratory illness, anemia, constipation, increased incidence of heart disease and cancer, low birth weights in infants and irritability.

Here is a review article about Canola Oil (rapeseed oil) and its toxic effects from a Swedish Medical Journal: Physiopathological effects of rapeseed oil: a review. ; Borg K; Acta Med Scand Suppl (1975) 585:5-13 ISSN: 0365-463X

Rapeseed oil has a growth retarding effect in animals. Some investigators claim that the high content of erucic acid in rapeseed oil alone causes this effect, while others consider the low ratio saturated/monounsaturated fatty acids in rapeseed oil to be a contributory factor. Normally erucic acid is not found or occurs in traces in body fat, but when the diet contains rapeseed oil erucic acid is found in depot fat, organ fat and milk fat. Erucic acid is metabolized in vivo to oleic acid. The effects of rapeseed oil on reproduction and adrenals, testes, ovaries, liver, spleen, kidneys, blood, heart and skeletal muscles have been investigated. Fatty infiltration in the heart muscle cells has been observed in the species investigated. In long-term experiments in rats erucic acid produces fibrosis of the myocardium. Erucic acid lowers the respiratory capacity of the heart mitochondria. The reduction of respiratory capacity is roughly proportional to the content of erucic acid in the diet, and diminishes on continued administration of erucic acid. The lifespan of rats is the same on corn oil, soybean oil, coconut oil, whale oil and rapeseed oil diet. Rats fed a diet with erucic acid or other docosenoic acids showed a lowered tolerance to cold stress (+ 4 degrees C). In Sweden erucic acid constituted 3-4% of the average intake of calories up to 1970 compared with about 0.4% at present.

What this study showed was that eating rapeseed oil (Canola Oil) causes the following damage:
1. Growth retardation
2. Damage to heart muscle
3. Lowered lung capacity
4. Lowered tolerance to cold temperatures

Generally rapeseed has a cumulative effect, taking almost 10 years before symptoms begin to manifest. It has a tendency to inhibit proper metabolism of foods and prohibits normal enzyme function. Canola is 4% Trans Fatty Acid, which has shown to have a direct link to cancer. These Trans Fatty acids are labeled as hydrogenated or partially hydrogenated oils. Avoid all of them!

According to John Thomas' book, Young Again, 12 years ago in England and Europe, rapeseed was fed to cows, pigs and sheep that later went blind and began attacking people. There were no further attacks after the rape seed was eliminated from their diet.

Source: David Dancu, N.D. http://www.karinya.com/canola.htm

Alkaline heating of canola and rapeseed meals reduces toxicity for chicks; Barrett JE,Klopfenstein CF, Leipold HW; Plant Foods Hum Nutr (1998) 52(1):9-15 ISSN: 0921-9668

Published Abstract: A simple method for improving the nutritive quality of canola and high glucosinolate rapeseed meals for monogastric animals (chicks) was developed; the meals were mixed with NaHCO3 and NH4HCO3, then heated in a conventional oven. Chicks fed untreated canola or rapeseed meals gained less weight than those fed a soybean meal diet, whereas chicks fed the alkaline heated meals had weight gains not significantly different than those fed the soybean diet. The antithyroid effect of the untreated rapeseed meal was reduced by alkaline treatment of the meals, as shown by improved T4 and free T4 levels in chicks fed the processed products. In chicks fed untreated or alkaline-treated canola or alkaline heated rapeseed meal, all thyroid hormone levels were similar to those of birds fed the soybean meal diet. However, heart tissue of chicks fed diets containing rapeseed or canola meals showed muscle fiber degeneration, although relative heart weights were the same in all groups. Liver tissue from most of the chicks in all dietary groups appeared normal or only slightly abnormal. The nutritive value of both rapeseed and canola meals was improved by this simple processing technique.
Department of Biology Kansas State University Manhattan USA.

This study shows that eating Canola oil depressed weight gain in the young, depression of thyroid function, and damaged heart muscle.

Effect of dietary cysteine supplements on canola meal toxicity and altered hepatic glutathione metabolism in the rat; Smith TK, Bray TM; J Anim Sci (1992 Aug) 70(8):2510-5 ISSN: 0021-8812

Published Abstract: Experiments were conducted to determine the effects of feeding canola meal (Brassica campestris and Brassica napus) on the rat hepatic glutathione detoxification system and whether dietary cysteine supplements might modify such effects. Rats were fed test diets for 14 d. Body weight change, feed consumption, hepatic glutathione concentration, and hepatic glutathione-Stransferase (GSHS-T) activities were determined. Weight gain was decreased when canola meal was fed, whereas hepatic glutathione concentrations increased, as did hepatic GSH-S-T activity. All effects correlated with total glucosinolate concentration in the canola meal. Dietary cysteine supplements, however, did not influence the growth reduction and increased hepatic glutathione concentrations caused by feeding canola meal. Supplemental cysteine prevented the elevation in hepatic GSH-S- T activity. The elevation in hepatic glutathione concentration caused by canola meals was not an overcompensation caused by an initial depletion and therefore reflected a general hepatotoxicity. Feeding supplemental cysteine increased hepatic glutathione levels at early time intervals and delayed the induction of GSH-S-T caused by canola meal toxicity. There was no beneficial effect of supplemental dietary cysteine in overcoming the toxicity of high levels of canola meal, but supplemental cysteine did modify the canola meal-induced changes in hepatic glutathione metabolism.

Department of Nutritional Sciences University of Guelph Ontario, Canada.

This study shows that eating Canola oil causes liver damage. It prevents the liver from detoxifying harmful things from the body.

Numerical density of cardiac myocytes in aged rats fed a cholesterol- rich diet and a canola oil diet (n-3 fatty acid rich); Aguila MB, Mandarim-de-Lacerda CA; Virchows Arch (1999 May) 434(5):451-3 ISSN: 0945-6317

Published Abstract: We studied the myocardium of 45 aged rats fed from 21 days after birth until 15 months of age with a standard rat diet (A) a cholesterol- rich diet (CHO) or canola oil (O). We analyzed the cardiac weight (CW) and, using unbiased stereological estimates, studied isotropic, uniform, random sections of the free left ventricular wall to determine the numerical density of the myocytes (NV[myocyte]). The Cardiac Weight was not statistically different between groups A and CHO: it was smallest in animals in group O (21.2% smaller in group O than in group A and 15.3% smaller in group O than in group CHO). NV[myocyte] was statistically different in all three groups and was greatest in animals in group O. By comparison with rats in group A, group CHO rats had an NV[myocyte] than was 51.3% smaller and group O, 33.3% greater. Aged rats fed with canola oil diet have a well-vascularized myocardium, which is probably associated with preservation of NV [myocyte] in the myocardium of these animals.

Laboratory of Morphometry and Cardiovascular Morphology State University of Rio de Janeiro, Brazil.

This study compared the size of hearts in rats fed one of three diets, a standard rat diet, a diet high in cholesterol and a diet high in Canola Oil. Those fed the Canola oil had the smallest hearts, supporting the previous study showing that Canola oil damages heart muscles.

Eating Fat and Obesity

The next issue is the belief that eating fat will make you fat. The truth is that eating Plastic Fat (trans fats, Canola Oil) makes you fat. If you make cell membranes from plastic fats, you will keep eating because your cells are starving even while they are coated with glucose that can't get into the cell. Also, eating Plastic Fats makes a liver that won't work leading to inability to manage your metabolism. Eating Plastic Fats makes a brain that can't control your endocrine system causing your thyroid, adrenals, pancreas, and gonads to malfunction. The paradox is that eating more good fat and stopping Plastic Fats causes you to become your normal weight.

To digest fat, you must have bile. The liver normally makes 1 1/2 quarts of bile per day. Because it makes so much, it needs a storage tank. That is the function of the gall bladder.

When you eat a fatty meal, the gall bladder must empty bile into the intestine to digest it. If you don't have enough bile, eating fat makes you nauseated. If your liver can't work well because it is made of plastic or is full of toxins, it can't make enough bile. If you have a gall bladder that is full of muddy debris because it rarely gets emptied or if your gall bladder is missing, you will not have enough bile to digest the fats you eat. As you can see, this becomes a vicious cycle. You can't repair your liver without eating and absorbing enough fat (about 0.1-0.2 pounds per day). You can't eat enough fat if you don't have enough bile because a lack of bile means you will be nauseated when you try to eat fat and even if you keep it down, you can't absorb it.

The secret is to take bile supplements with each meal until your liver is repaired enough to make bile normally. You can get "Ox Bile" at most health food stores. If you don't have a gall bladder, you must take bile supplements with every meal the rest of your life or you won't be able to make normal cells. That means you will be sick.

Measuring Cell Membranes

We can measure the function of cell membranes using a device called the Biological Impedance Analysis device (BIA). This device is in widespread use in every physiology department in the world. It gives us a measurement called "Phase Angle" that can suggest to us if you are made of

Biological Impedance Analysis (BIA)

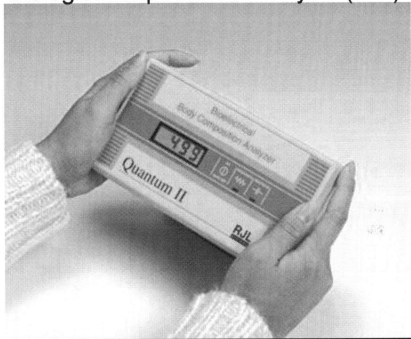

http://www.rjlsystems.com/products/

ATP/ADP

We have been discussing the storage of electrons by the cells. We have discussed how cell membranes are primary capacitors to store electrons for use by the cells. This voltage is used primarily to control the electronic circuitry of the cell membrane since it functions as a semi-conductor, a diode, a transistor, and a microprocessor.

Inside the cell, we have another electron storage system known as ATP/ADP. This rechargeable battery system is

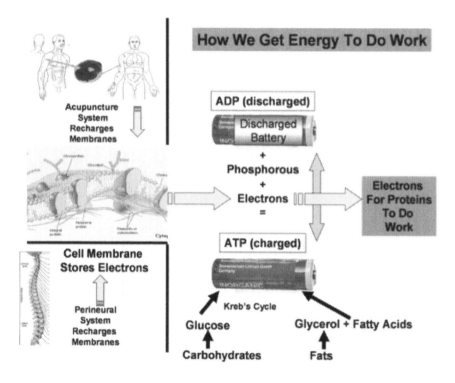

used to make many of the cell's chemical functions work.

Remember that when oxygen is available, we make 38 molecules of ATP from one unit of fatty acids, but when oxygen is unavailable, we only make two! This inability to provide electrons for critical chemical pathways of the cell is part of chronic illness.

How Are Electrons Moved From Place to Place in the Body?

Fibrous tissue has the least impedance or resistance to the flow of electrons of any tissue in the body. Therefore, wherever you find fibrous tissue in the body, inserting two functions. One is structural. It is providing support for the adjacent tissue. The second function, however, is to move electrons from place to place.

The human body has two wiring systems. Both are made of fibrous tissue. One is the fibrous encasement of nerves that Robert Becker named the "analog perineural nervous system". The other is the acupuncture system.

Analog Perineural Nervous System

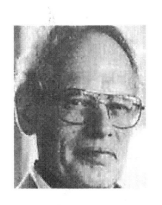

Robert Becker was an orthopedic surgeon. His classic book The Body Electric is a must-read for everyone interested in healing. He became interested in the fact that in the human if you lose a piece of bone, you will make more bone. If you lose a piece of any other tissue, it is replaced by scar tissue. In the human, it was believed that only bone is capable of regeneration. We now know that all tissue can regenerate with the proper conditions.

Regeneration is the ability of lower animals to replace missing body parts. It is particularly evident in the salamander. For this reason, Becker decided to study regeneration in the salamander.

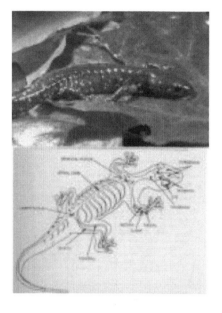

The salamander has essentially the same anatomy as the human = same number of bones, muscles, and nerves in the same arrangement.

The salamander is capable of growing an exact replacement of an arm, leg, eye, ear, up to 1/3 of its brain, almost all of its digestive tract, and up to 1/2 of its heart. If you poke out a salamander's eye, he simply grows a new one. If you cut off his arm, he simply grows another one. The question is, "Why can the salamander grow new parts when we can't?"

The salamander is so efficient at regeneration that it does not get cancer! The regeneration of the salamander cannot be explained by the chemical-mechanistic views of traditional medicine.

To study regeneration, Becker would amputate the arm of the salamander. He found that the stump would become electropositive (electron stealer) of about +25 mV, and he called this the "Current of Injury". The skin would grow over the stump. The cut ends of nerves in the stump would connect with each skin cell called neuroepithelial junction (NEJ).

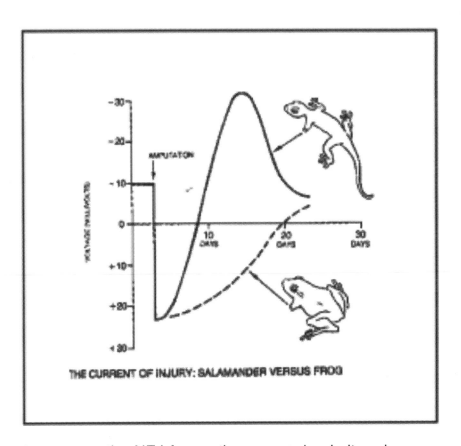

THE CURRENT OF INJURY: SALAMANDER VERSUS FROG

As soon as the NEJ forms, the reversed polarity changes normal cells to adult stem cells that had been named "blastema" by Thomas Hunt Morgan. This mass of primitive cells that appears between cut end of the stump and the NEJ (blastema or stem cells) are primitive cells from bone, muscle, etc. that have de-differentiated back to the embryonic state. As soon as they form, the voltage goes to −30 mV (electron donor).

Becker found that if he removed and re-implanted the blastema before ten days, it grows a duplicate of the organ it is near. For example, if he amputated an arm, made a slit near the salamander's tail and implanted it, a new second tail would grow. If he implanted it near the hind leg, the

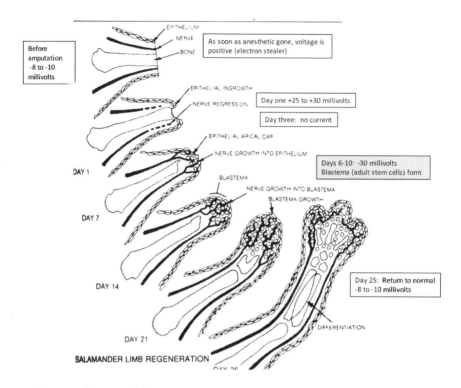

Before amputation -8 to -10 millivolts

EPITHELIUM
NERVE
BONE
As soon as anesthetic gone, voltage is positive (electron stealer)

EPITHELIAL INGROWTH
NERVE REGRESSION
Day one +25 to +30 millivolts
Day three: no current

EPITHELIAL APICAL CAP
NERVE GROWTH INTO EPITHELIUM
Days 6-10: -30 millivolts
Blastema (adult stem cells) form

DAY 1

BLASTEMA
NERVE GROWTH INTO BLASTEMA
BLASTEMA GROWTH

DAY 7

DAY 14
Day 25: Return to normal -8 to -10 millivolts

DIFFERENTIATION
DAY 21

SALAMANDER LIMB REGENERATION
DAY 28

salamander would grow a second hind leg.

Then he found something else unusual. If he removed and re-implanted the blastema after ten days, it grows a duplicate of the organ it is from. For example, if he amputated an arm but waited more than ten days after the blastema formed to remove and implant it near the tail, it grew an arm out of the tail area instead of another tail. Thus the blastema was being programmed what it was to become during the first ten days.

Becker wondered how the blastema was being programmed and assumed it was the nervous system. He then cut the nerves going to the arm and then amputated the arm. To his surprise, nothing changed. Harvesting and re-implanting the blastema before ten days grew a local organ and after ten days grew the same organ or limb) that was amputated. He couldn't figure out how it was being programmed.

He then made one millimeter sections of the area and found that the nerves were not growing back into the stem cells, but the fibrous tissue around the nerves were quickly growing into the stem cells (blastema). These fibrous cells were carrying the information to program the blastema.

Becker went on to discover that we have an entire second nervous system made of fibrous tissue surrounding our nerve.

He named this the "Analog Perineural Nervous System". The nerve-impulse nerves of the brain and body are digital. That means that information is in discrete steps of on/off. It is sensitive to the frequency of the signal. It controls the conscious mind and the autonomic nervous system (automatic control of blood pressure, breathing, etc.)

The second nervous system of the body is the perineural system of glial cells, Schwann cells, etc. that surround the other nerves. It is an analog system = continuously variable strength of signal, direction of flow, and waves of strength. It controls growth, healing, and biological cycles.

Where we have always thought that the fibrous tissue of the body serves only as structural support, Becker and Nördenstrom have shown that fibrous tissue in the body also serves to conduct electrons, much like copper wire in our homes.

It seems that Becker never realized that the fibrous sheath called the perineural nervous system was actually bringing in electrons to change the voltage from operating voltage to healing voltage.

The analog perineural system:

1. Delivers the information to the blastema about how to grow a new body part (regeneration). Nerves have nothing to do with it.
2. Senses injury and controls repair.
3. Controls local environments.
4. Is the primary system in the brain.
5. Regulates our consciousness.
6. Regulates decision making.

Most scientists do not believe that cells can dedifferentiate from normal cells back to adult stem cells. It is believed that once cells differentiate into functional cells, they cannot go back the other way. For example, once a stem cell becomes a liver cell, can never be anything except a liver cell. Becker showed that isn't true. Frog red blood cells have a nucleus. Becker exposed them to small electron-stealer currents in billionths of amperes). They became stem cells.

When cells differentiate into cells in organs, genes that are not needed are turned off. However, they are still present. With the proper voltage, these genes can be switched back on as the cell de-differentiates back into adult stem cells.

Vertebra	Areas Supplied by Nerves	Possible Effects or Conditions
C1	Blood supply to the head, pituitary, scalp, bones of the face, brain, inner and middle ear, sympathetic nervous system.	Headache, nervousness, insomnia, head colds, high blood pressure, migraines, mental conditions, nervous breakdowns, amnesia, epilepsy, chronic tiredness.
C2	Eyes, optic nerve, auditory nerve, sinuses, mastoid bones, tongue, forehead	Sinus trouble, allergies, crossed eyes, deafness, eye trouble, earache, fainting spells, blindness.
C3	Cheeks, outer ear, facial bones, teeth, facial nerve	Neuralgia, tinnitus, acne, eczema
C4	Nose, lips, mouth, Eustachian tubes, mucous membranes	Hay fever, hearing loss, post-nasal drip.
C5	Vocal cords, neck lymph glands, pharynx	Laryngitis, hoarseness, sore throat
C6	Neck muscles, shoulders, tonsils	Stiff neck, pain in upper arm, tonsillitis, whooping cough, croup
C7	Thyroid gland, bursae in shoulders, elbows	Bursitis, colds, thyroid conditions, goiter, tennis elbow, tendonitis

T1	Arms from elbows down, hands, wrists, fingers, esophagus, trachea	Asthma, cough, difficult breathing, shortness of breath, pain in lower arms and hands, carpal tunnel syndrome.
T2	Heart, pericardium, valves, arteries	Heart conditions, angina
T3	Lungs, bronchial tubes, pleura, chest, breast, nipples	Bronchitis, pleuritis, pneumonia, congestion, influenza, grip
T4	Gall Bladder and common duct	Gall bladder pain, jaundice, shingles
T5	Liver, solar plexus, blood	Liver conditions, low blood pressure, anemia, poor circulation, arthritis
T6	Stomach	Indigestion, heartburn, dyspepsia
T7	Pancreas, Islets of Langerhans, duodenum	Diabetes, ulcers, gastritis, hypoglycemia
T8	Spleen, diaphragm	Weakened immune system, acute and chronic infections, hiccoughs
T9	Adrenals	Allergies, hives, hypertension, anemia, hypoglycemia, obesity, hair loss.

T10	Kidneys	Kidney stones, arteriosclerosis, chronic fatigue, nephritis, kidney infections
T11	Kidneys, ureters	Skin conditions like acne or pimples, boils, autoimmune diseases
T12	Small intestine, fallopian tubes, lymph, circulation	Joint pain, gas pain, bloating
L1	Large intestine, inguinal rings	Constipation, colitis, dysentery, diarrhea, hernias
L2	Appendix, abdomen, upper leg	Appendicitis, cramps, acidosis, varicose veins
L3	Sex organs, ovaries, testicles, uterus, bladder, knee	Bladder troubles, menstrual trouble, miscarriages, bed wetting, incontinence, menopausal symptoms, knee pain
L4	Prostate gland, low back muscles, sciatic nerve	Sciatica, low back pain, painful & frequent urination, backaches
L5	Lower legs, ankle, feet, toes, arteries	Poor circulation in legs, swollen ankles, cold feet, weakness in legs, leg cramps

The easiest way to access the perineural nervous system is at the spine. In the chart, you can see where each autonomic nerve exits the spine and which organs are connected to each nerve. One can use an electronic device such as the Tennant BioModulator to tap into any of these wires to measure the voltage of the connected organ or to send electrons to that organ.

The Acupuncture System

One of the body' wiring systems is the analog perineural nervous system. The other is the acupuncture system. Remember that both wiring systems are made of fibrous tissue.

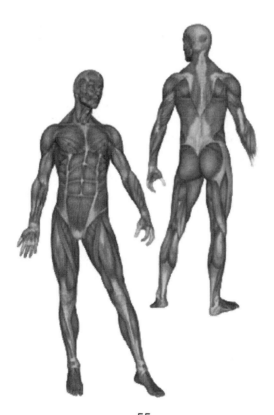

A sheath or cable made of fibrous tissue is called fascia. Fascia interpenetrates and surrounds muscles, bones, organs, nerves, blood vessels and other structures. Fascia is an uninterrupted, three-dimensional web of tissue that extends from head to toe, from front to back, from interior to exterior.

I encourage you to go back and read the section about semiconductors, diodes, transistors, and microprocessors.

The fascia of the body are semiconductors, diodes, transistors, and microprocessors. These connect with and communicate with the cells of each organ.

Remember that one of the characteristics of semiconductors is that electrons moved in only one direction. This becomes important when considering how acupuncture meridian's work.

In the images you will notice that fascia surround each muscle, connect with a fascial sheath that surrounds each organ, and then small fibers connect the sheets around each organ down to each little cluster of cells. In this way, each cell of the body is wired to the common wire that goes up the center of the back and down the center of the front of the body. This is the acupuncture system.

Helene Langevin, M.D. is a research assistant professor of neurology at the University of Vermont School of Medicine. She and her colleagues published a seminal article about acupuncture meridians:

The Anatomical Record, Volume 269, Issue 6, 2002, pp. 257-265. Relationship Of Acupuncture Points And Meridians To Connective Tissue Planes. Helene M. Langevin,* Jason A. Yandow.

Acupuncture meridians traditionally are believed to constitute channels connecting the surface of the body to internal organs. We hypothesize that the network of acupuncture points and meridians can be viewed as a representation of the network formed by interstitial connective tissue.

This hypothesis is supported by ultrasound images showing connective tissue cleavage planes at acupuncture points in normal human subjects. To test this hypothesis, we mapped acupuncture points in serial gross anatomical sections through the human arm.

We found an 80% correspondence between the sites of acupuncture points and the location of inter-muscular or intramuscular connective tissue planes in postmortem tissue sections.

We propose that the anatomical relationship of acupuncture points and meridians to connective tissue planes is relevant to acupuncture's mechanism of action and suggests a potentially important integrative role for interstitial connective tissue.

Thus Langevin and her colleagues have shown us that the acupuncture system is essentially the fascial planes of the body.

Remember that the fascia are made of fibrous tissue. Remember also that fibrous tissue has the least resistance to the flow of electrons through the body. Remember also that this tissue is an electronic semiconductor, diode, etc.

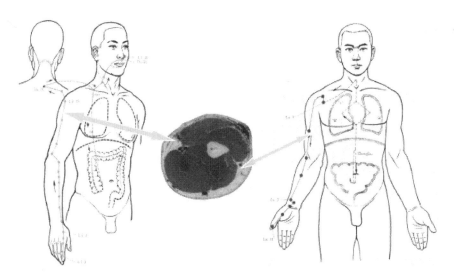

In the graphic you can see the cross section of an arm. You can also see the classical drawings for the lung and large intestine meridians. You can see in the cross-section the fascial wires in the arm that are at the fibrous wires known as the lung and large intestine meridians.

Ionic Transfer Of Electrons

Besides the two wiring systems of the body (the perineural system and the acupuncture system) there is an additional means of moving electrons from place to place. There is an ionic transfer within the blood plasma. This was eloquently described by Björn Nördenstrom   in his classical book Biologically Closed Electric Circuits.

In summary, we see there are three ways in which electrons are moved from place to place. One is by way of the wiring system known as the perineural nervous system. The second is by way of the wiring system known as the acupuncture meridian system. The third is ionically within the blood plasma.

How Do We Measure the Voltage in Organs?

It is difficult to use a voltmeter to measure the voltage in organs via the perineural nervous system or the acupuncture system. Voltage in the body pulses. Thus when you use a voltmeter, it will give a wide range of readings. It usually starts high and then, over a few minutes, it settles down to a more constant reading. Therefore it is common to use an ohmmeter to measure the voltage and then convert that to volts using Ohm's Law. That says that Voltage = ohms x amps. If one assumes that amperage is constant, then ohms = voltage.

One can also use the Assess Mode of the Tennant BioModulator to estimate the voltage.

One can measure the voltage of organs by using the perineural nervous system or the acupuncture system.

If one wants to use the perineural system, you can use the chart displayed above to know what organ corresponds to which vertebra.

The acupuncture system is more difficult for most to understand.   Its origins are over 5000 years ago---long before there was a clear understanding of anatomy and physiology.   For example, there is no brain or nervous system in acupuncture theory.

Another system that is over 5000 years old is the Vedas and the concept of chakras.   In this system it is believed that there are energy spheres in the body that connect to the universe.   When these energy spheres, called chakras, are spinning incorrectly, disease results.

Chakras, as described above, are energy centers along the spine located at major branchings of the human nervous system, beginning at the base of the spinal column and moving upward to the top of the skull.

"Chakras are considered to be a point or nexus of biophysical energy or prana of the human body. Shumsky states that "prana is the basic component of your subtle body, your energy field, and the entire chakra system...the key to life and source of energy in the universe."

The following seven primary chakras are commonly described:

- Muladhara (Sanskrit: Mūlādhāra) Base or Root Chakra (last bone in spinal cord *coccyx*)
- Swadhisthana (Sanskrit: Svādhiṣṭhāna) Sacral Chakra (ovaries/prostate)
- Manipura (Sanskrit: Maṇipūra) Solar Plexus Chakra (navel area)
- Anahata (Sanskrit: Anāhata) Heart Chakra (heart area)
- Vishuddha (Sanskrit: Viśuddha) Throat Chakra (throat and neck area)
- Ajna (Sanskrit: Ājñā) Brow or Third Eye Chakra (pineal gland or third eye)
- Sahasrara (Sanskrit: Sahasrāra) Crown Chakra (Top of the head; 'Soft spot' of a newborn)"
www.wikipedia.com

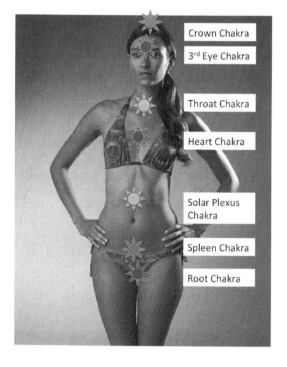

Another system of energy distribution was developed by Master Jiro Murai, a Japanese gentleman about to die in 1912. It is said that he went into a deep sleep and awoke well with the knowledge of how to balance energy in the body. Others report that he remembered a technique he was taught as a child and applied this to

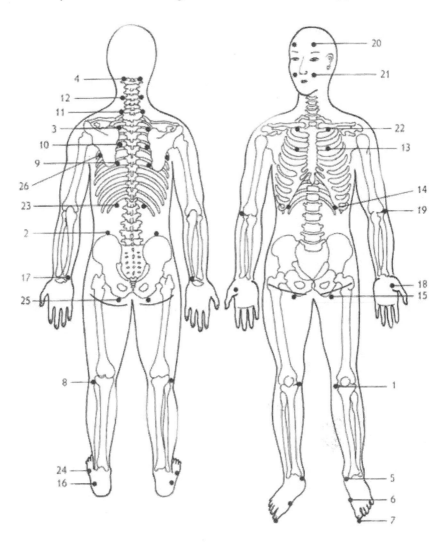

himself only to find himself cured in one week.

The system is called Jin Shin or Jin Shin Jyutsu. The system consists of the therapist placing both hands on certain spots in a series of protocols to correct the flow of energy.

It is said that Jiro Murai taught Haruki Kato, MD this method. Apparently Kato and Murai taught Mary Mariko Iino-Burmeister the techniques. Mary, a Japanese American, returned to California and began teaching the techniques there and later in Arizona.

The graphic depicts the points used by Burmeister in her teachings and their acupuncture correspondences. In the Murai technique, the points are listed as a number. For example, you might use your hands to connect right #4 with right #20. This would be the same as connecting GB-20 and GB-14 in acupuncture terminology.

In the 1990's, Glenn King, PhD of Dallas TX sought to learn and understand Murai's system. He studied the methods taught by Mary Burmeister. He eventually was given copies of Murai's drawings that were originally given to Mary Burmeister. His interpretation of the system differed from Burmeister's. He eventually developed a system called "The King Method" or TKM. Although I have been trained by him in his system, he strongly enforces his copyrights to the material. Since it is difficult to know what material is Murai's or more ancient and not covered by copyright and what is King's version, it is difficult to discuss his system.

I found it difficult to believe that the body contained different systems that were not working together. As I continued to study various acupuncture texts, it became apparent to me that there were spots on the primary acupuncture circuits (governor and conception meridians) where multiple meridians crossed. These points corresponded closely to the locations described for many of the chakras.

Understanding that the acupuncture system is the same as the fascial system, I noted that the location of crossing points of the fascia were the same as some of the Jin Shin/Murai points.

Further examination of these facts led to the understanding that there is a primary cable that carries voltage up the back and down the front of the body. Also, there is a central terminal for each region of the body on that cable that sends voltage to every organ in that region. For example, there are points on the front and back of the skull that send voltage first to the right and left of the skull and then to each organ in

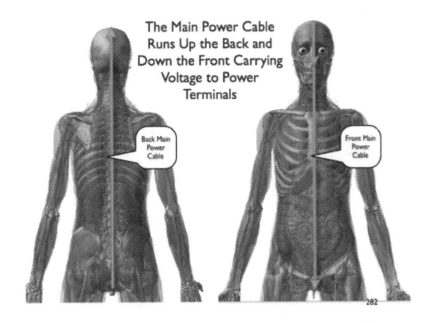

the skull. The central terminal corresponds to what is classically called the third eye chakra. The lateral terminals correspond to what the Jin Shin/Murai system calls Energy Spheres #20 and acupuncture calls gall bladder 14 (GB-14).

I began to call these switching points on the primary meridians "Switching Terminals" or "BioTerminals®". I felt they needed a different name because they are close to, but not the same as, chakra positions.

Conception Meridian	Terminals	BioTerminals
CV-1	CV, GV, Penetrating	Primary = Root
CV-2	CV, LV	
CV-3	CV, SP, LV, KI	Pelvis BioTerminal
CV-4	CV, SP, LV, KI	
CV-7	CV, KI	
CV-10	CV, SP	
CV-12	CV, SI, TB, ST	Abdomen BioTerminal
CV-13	CV, ST, SI	
CV-15	Luo Points	Xiphoid
CV-17	CV, SP, KI, SI, TB	Chest BioTerminal
CV-22	CV, Yin Linking	Throat BioTerminal
CV-24	CV, GV, LI, ST	Chin

Governor Meridian	Location	Terminals	BioTerminal
GV-1	Coccyx to Anus	Luo Points, GV, CV, GB, KI	Primary = Root

GV-4	L-2/KI		Pelvic BioTerminal
GV-6	T-11./SP		Abdomen BioTerminal
G-11	T-5/HT		Chest BioTerminal
GV-13	T-1	GV, BL	Throat BioTerminal
GV-14	C-7	GV, Six Yang Channels	Throat BioTerminal
GV-15	C-2	GV, Yang Linking Vessel	Skull BioTerminal
GV-16	C-1	GV, Yang Linking Vessel	Skull BioTerminal
GV-17		GV, BL	
GV-20		GV, BL, GB, TB, LV	Crown BioTerminal
GV-24		GV, BL, ST	
GV-26		GV, LI, ST	Upper Lip

The lateral BioTerminals are shown in the graphic. Notice that we have a central and right and left lateral BioTerminals for the head, neck/upper chest, chest, abdomen, and pelvis.

Lateral Terminals

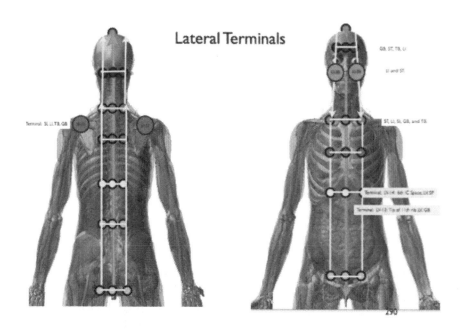

Look at the similarities between the BioTerminals and the

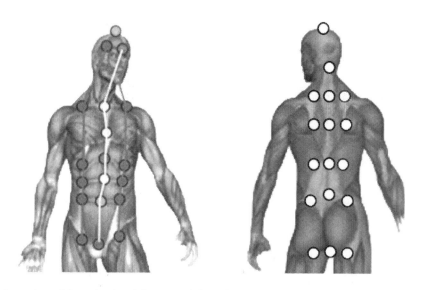

bands of fascia in this graphic. The lateral BioTerminals are very similar to the Jin Shin Points.

Now we have an easy way to determine the voltages of the organs in each region of the body. Let's say that you have pneumonia. You will certainly have low voltage in the chest BioTerminal®. It may be front or back or both. If you have stomach ulcers, you will have low voltage in the abdomen

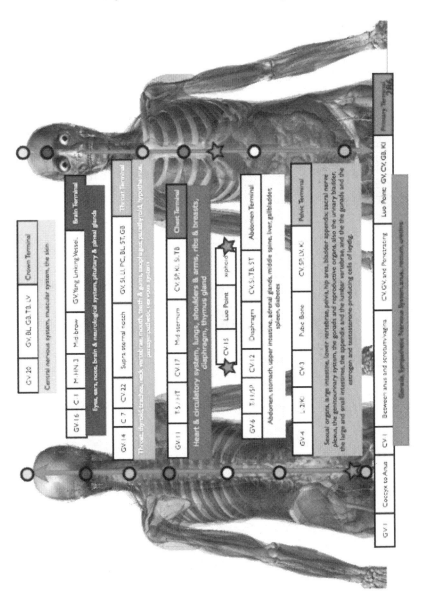

BioTerminal®. It can be on the left or the right or both.

The locations of these BioTerminals are noted above. The head BioTerminal® is between the brows on the front and at C-1 on the back. The neck BioTerminal® is at the supra-sternal notch in the front and at C-7 on the back. The chest BioTerminal® is at the mid-sternum in the front and at T-5 in the back. The abdomen BioTerminal® is halfway between the bottom of the sternum and the umbilicus on the front and at T-11 on the back. The pelvic BioTerminal® is just above the pubic bone on the front and at L-2 on the back.

There is also a BioTerminal® on the top of the skull and in the perineum. It can be measured over the coccyx.

Note Similarities to Kabbalah

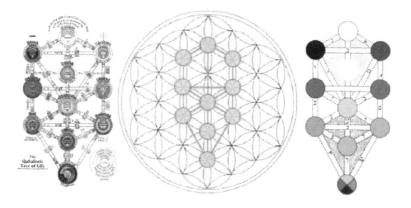

291

Note that the BioTerminal System has some similarities to the Kabbalah's Tree of Life. It also describes energetic pathways.

There is a safety circuit that connects the main cables in case one gets shorted out. It runs from the bottom of the sternum (xiphoid) to the coccyx. It is shown as a star in the graphic. This safety circuit often is necessary after abdominal surgery creates a scar that shorts out the normal flow of electrons through the main cables. You can see how the electrons normally flow up the back and down the front. Now imagine a scar on your abdomen from surgery or an

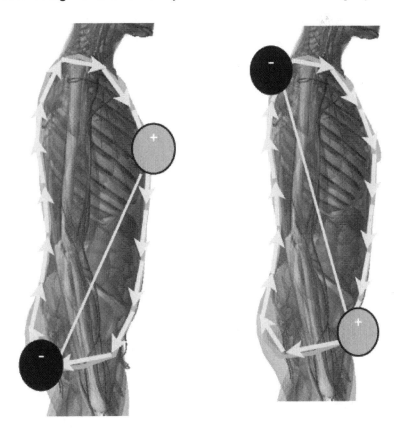

injury. It would short out the circuit. The body's defense

against this is to use the "detour" from the xiphoid (bottom of sternum) to the coccyx. This protects the vital brain and heart, but it would leave the pelvis organs with reduced voltage, resulting in pelvic disorders. To overcome this, there is another "detour" from C-7 to the supra-pubic BioTerminal®. This allows some electrons to flow from C-7 to the pelvis to overcome blockages.

It is unfortunate that surgeons know nothing about the serious side effects of scars on the normal flow of electrons to organs via the acupuncture system of fascia.

One should treat scars with topical iodine and the Tennant BioModulator to reduce their shorting effect on the flow of electrons.

The Organs of the Body are Wired Together as Tesla Circuits.

The father of electricity was Nikola Tesla. He had a much more dramatic influence on electronic devices and the delivery of electricity than Thomas Edison.

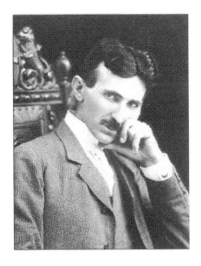

Nikola Tesla (10 July 1856 – 7 January 1943) was an inventor and a mechanical and electrical engineer. He was one of the most important contributors to the birth of commercial electricity and is best known for his many revolutionary developments in the field of electromagnetism in the late 19th and early 20th centuries. Tesla's patents and theoretical work formed the basis of modern alternating current (AC) electrical power systems, including the polyphase system of electrical distribution and the AC motor, with which he helped usher in the Second Industrial Revolution. www.wikipedia.

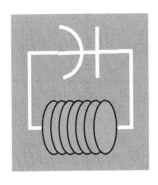

In 1895, Tesla invented the Tuned Circuit or Resonating Circuit. It consists of a coil wired to a capacitor. When they are wired on a box-shaped circuit, it is called "wired in parallel". Parallel Tuned Circuits are used in radio and other electronics to couple resonate energy from one circuit to another in transmitters and receivers.

In acupuncture theory, half of the organs are said to be yin organs and half are said to be yang organs. A yin organ is always connected to a yang organ.

It became apparent to me that the yin organs are capacitors and the yang organs are hollow organs that serve as coils. They are wired together through

Capacitors	Yin	Coils	Yang
Governor Meridian	GV	Conception Meridian	CV
Lung	LU	Large Intestine	LI
Pericardium	PC	Triple Burner or Sanjiao	TB
Heart	HI	Small Intestine	SI
Liver	LV	Gall Bladder	GB
Spleen	SP	Stomach	ST

connecting meridians to form Tesla Resonating Circuits.

The yin organs (capacitors; solid organs) are all wired to the Main Cable that runs up the back. The yang organs (coils; hollow organs) are all wired to the Main Cable that runs down the front of the body.

The thing that is confusing at first is that the wires that form the Tesla Resonating Circuits with each organ pain make a loop through either an arm or a leg. The loop also passes through a BioTerminal®. Where the loops connect in the arms or legs are called the Luo Points in acupuncture theory.

Point	Connected Meridians
LU-6	Lung Meridian
LU-7	Large Intestine Meridian

PC-8	Triple Burner (Sanjiao)
TB-5	Pericardium Meridian
SI-7	Heart Meridian
HT-5	Small Intestine Meridian
BL-58	Kidney Meridian
KI-4	Bladder Meridian
GB-37	Liver Meridian
LV-5	Gall Bladder
ST-40	Spleen Meridian
SP-4	Stomach Meridian

One circuit that is unique is the liver/gall bladder circuit. It controls the entire Main Cable System and is thus critical in the function of the entire system.

There are two unusual names in acupuncture theory that are used in the same way the names of organs are used, but they are not organs. The names are "Triple Burner" or "Triple Heater" or "Sanjiao". These names are synonyms. The other unusual circuit is called the "Pericardium" although it has very little to do with the covering of the heart. The Triple Burner is part of the yang or hollow circuitry and the Pericardium is part of the yin or capacitor circuitry.

The Triple Burner is wired to the front BioTerminal of the skull and the Pericardium is wired to the back BioTerminal of the skull.

The Large Intestine circuit is wired to the front Neck BioTerminal and the Lung circuit is wired to the back Neck BioTerminal.

The Small Intestine circuit is wired to the front Chest BioTerminal and the Heart circuit is wired to the back Chest BioTerminal.

The Stomach circuit is wired to the front Abdominal BioTerminal and the Spleen circuit is wired to the back Abdominal BioTerminal.

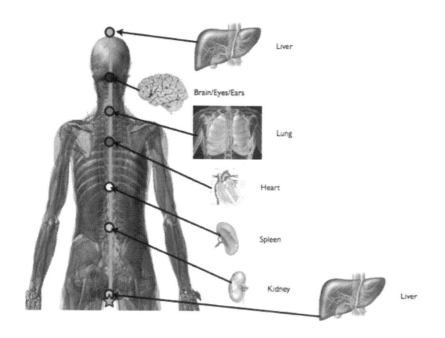

The Bladder circuit is wired to the front Pelvis BioTerminal and the Kidney circuit is wired to the back Pelvis BioTerminal.

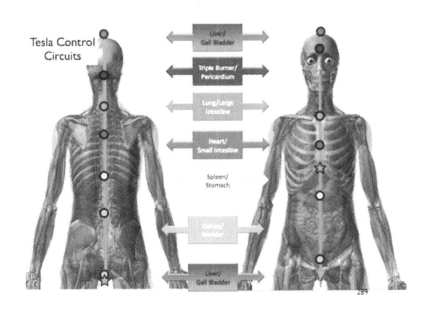

Tesla Control Circuits

Liver/ Gall Bladder	
Triple Burner/ Pericardium	
Lung/Large Intestine	
Heart/ Small Intestine	
Spleen/ Stomach	
Kidney/ Bladder	
Liver/ Gall Bladder	

289

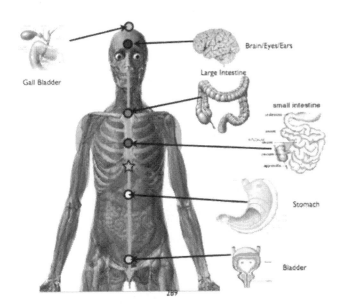

Gall Bladder

Brain/Eyes/Ears

Large Intestine

small intestine

Stomach

Bladder

259

The Liver circuit is wired to the Crown BioTerminal and the Gall Bladder circuit is wired to the Base or Root BioTerminal.

Remember that the Liver circuit connects to the Crown BioTerminal and the Gall Bladder circuit connects to the Root or Base BioTerminal. I prefer to use the liver and gall bladder points on the knees instead of the classical Luo points for these circuits.

Remember that Tesla Circuits are designed to measure and adjust other circuits.

When a BioTerminal's voltage begins to drop, that is recognized by the associated Tesla Circuit. It moves electrons from the arm or leg muscles to the BioTerminal in an effort to modulate it back to normal. Thus it is important to exercise to keep the arm and leg muscle batteries charged.

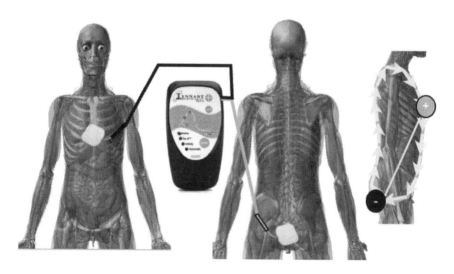

When the total body voltage is low, you can use the Tennant BioModulator as a portable battery charger while you are correcting the reasons for the low voltage. Place a patch over the supra-pubic BioTerminal and one over C-7. Attach the wire to the Tennant BioModulator and run it 24 hours per

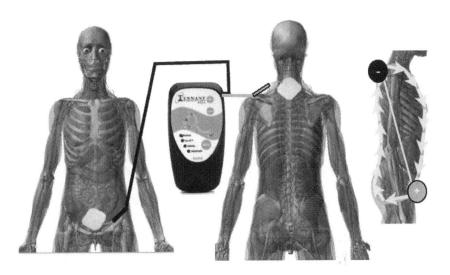

day until your voltages are normal.

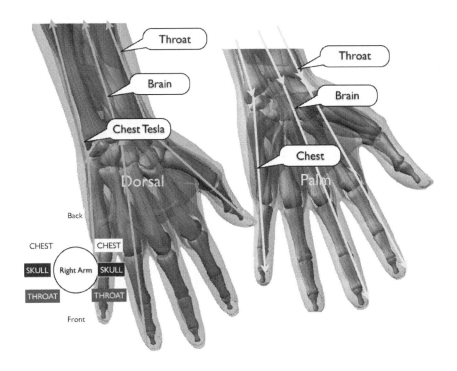

The supra-pubic BioTerminal controls all of the yin organs (capacitors, solid organs). The BioTerminal at C-7 controls

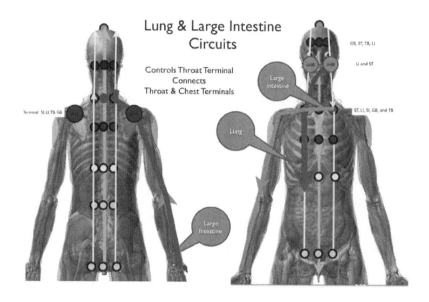

all the yang organs (hollow, coil organs).

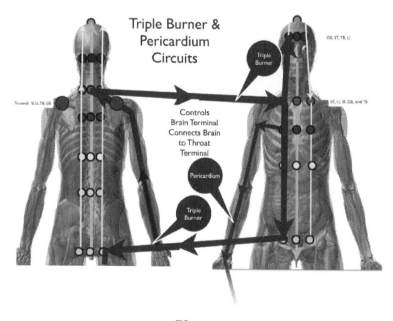

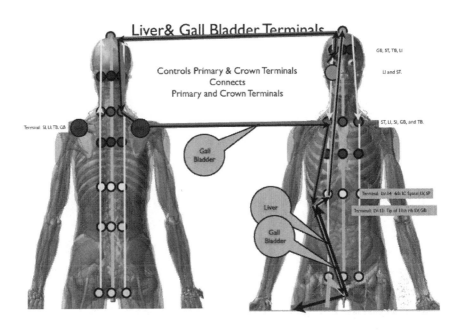

Liver & Gall Bladder Terminals

Controls Primary & Crown Terminals
Connects
Primary and Crown Terminals

GB, ST, TB, LI

LI and ST.

ST, LI, SI, GB, and TB.

Terminal: SI, LI, TB, GB

Gall Bladder

Liver

Gall Bladder

Terminal: Lv 14: 4th IC Space; LV, SP

Terminal: LV-13: Tip of 11th rib LV, GB

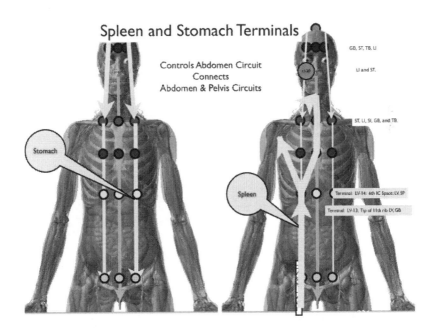

Spleen and Stomach Terminals

Controls Abdomen Circuit
Connects
Abdomen & Pelvis Circuits

GB, ST, TB, LI

LI and ST.

ST, LI, SI, GB, and TB.

Stomach

Spleen

Terminal: LV-14: 4th IC Space; LV, SP

Terminal: LV-13: Tip of 11th rib LV, GB

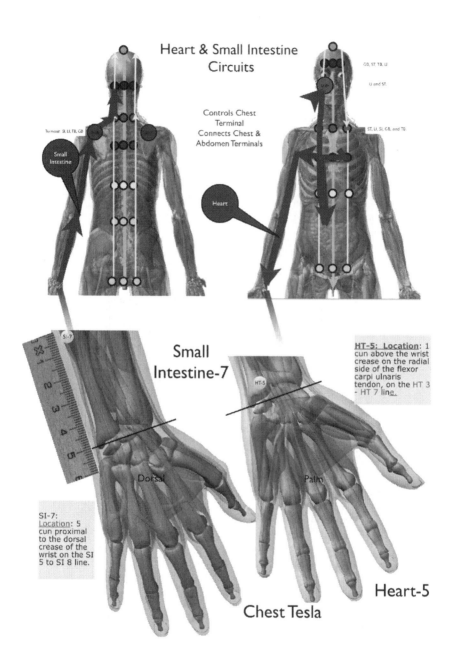

Heart & Small Intestine Circuits

Controls Chest
Terminal
Connects Chest &
Abdomen Terminals

GB, ST, TB, LI

LI and ST

Small
Intestine

Terminal: SI, LI, TB, GB

ST, LI, SI, GB, and TB

Heart

Small Intestine-7

SI-7
HT-5: Location: 1 cun above the wrist crease on the radial side of the flexor carpi ulnaris tendon, on the HT 3 - HT 7 line.

HT-5

Dorsal

Palm

SI-7:
Location: 5 cun proximal to the dorsal crease of the wrist on the SI 5 to SI 8 line.

Heart-5

Chest Tesla

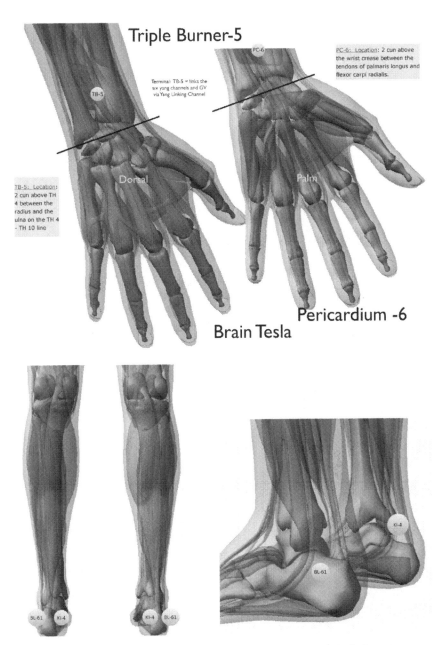

Triple Burner-5

PC-6

PC-6: Location: 2 cun above the wrist crease between the tendons of palmaris longus and flexor carpi radialis.

Terminal: TB-5 = links the six yang channels and GV via Yang Linking Channel

TB-5

TB-5: Location: 2 cun above TH 4 between the radius and the ulna on the TH 4 - TH 10 line

Dorsal

Palm

Pericardium -6

Brain Tesla

BL-61

KI-4

KI-4

BL-61

BL-61

KI-4

KI-4

BL-61

Pelvis Tesla

KI-4: On the anterior border of the Achilles Tendon

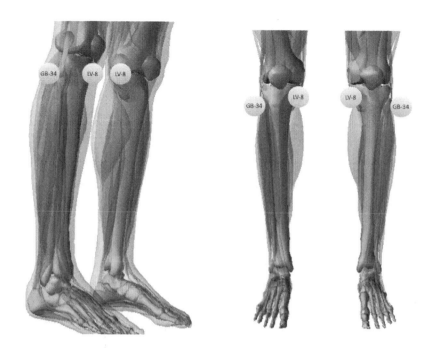

Crown/Base Tesla

Five Element vs. Six Element Theories

In classical acupuncture theory, there is a system called the "Five Element Theory"

"The Wu Xing or the Five Movements, Five Phases or Five Steps/Stages, are chiefly an ancient mnemonic device, in many traditional Chinese fields.

It is sometimes translated as Five Elements, but the Wu Xing are chiefly an ancient mnemonic device, hence the preferred translation of "movements", "phases" or "steps" over "elements". By the same token, Mu is thought of as "Tree" rather than "Wood".

The five elements are:

1. Wood = Liver and Gall Bladder
2. Fire = Heart and Small Intestine
3. Earth = Spleen and Stomach
4. Metal = Lung and Large Intestine
5. Water = Kidney and Bladder

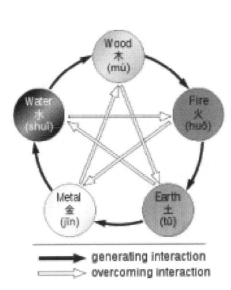

generating interaction
overcoming interaction

The system of five phases was used for describing interactions and relationships between phenomena. It was employed as a device in many fields of early Chinese thought, including seemingly disparate fields such as geomancy or Feng shui, astrology, traditional Chinese medicine, music, military strategy and martial arts."

The common memory jogs, which help to remind in what order the phases are:
1. Wood feeds Fire; (liver supports heart)
2. Fire creates Earth (ash); (heart supports spleen)
3. Earth bears Metal; (spleen supports lung)
4. Metal carries Water (as in a bucket or tap, or water condenses on metal); (lung supports kidney)
5. Water nourishes Wood." (kidney supports liver)

It also supposes that there is opposition.
1. Wood absorbs Water; (liver steals from kidney)

2. Water rusts Metal; (kidney steals from lung)
3. Metal breaks up Earth; (lung steals from spleen)
4. Earth smothers Fire; (spleen steals from heart)
5. Fire burns Wood. (heart steals from liver)
www.wikipedia.com

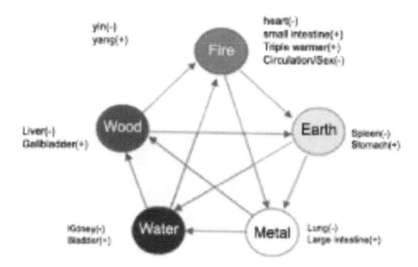

This concept becomes more understandable than simply watching what happens around you if you look at the way electrons flow through the acupuncture system.

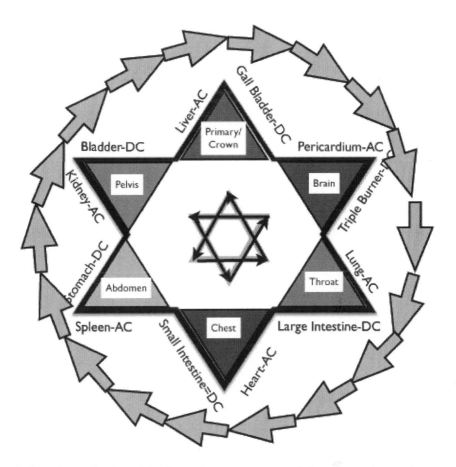

I developed what I believe is a more useful system based on a six-pointed star instead of a five star (element) theory. Start with the bladder Tesla at the posterior Pelvic BioTerminal. It goes up the Main Cable to the Primary or Crown BioTerminal via the Liver and Gall Bladder Tesla. This then connects with the Brain BioTerminal via the Pericardium and Triple Burner Tesla circuits. This leads us to the Throat BioTerminal via the Lung and Large Intestine Tesla. You can continue to follow the circuits in the graphic above.

If one of the BioTerminals is blocked---say by a scar---it backs up the flow of electrons to the one before it and, to some degree, to the one before that. The "detour" circuits noted above can ameliorate this to some degree.

When finding low or high voltage in the BioTerminal circuits, you must look to see if the blockage of a BioTerminal is causing higher voltage in the BioTerminal before it and lower voltage in the BioTerminal(s) after it. If so, you will want to be sure there isn't a scar blocking the forward movement of electrons and open the BioTerminal in front of the one in question, then amplify the one behind it and finally open the one that is the problem. It's like driving a car. You can't move forward if the car in front of you is stalled even if the

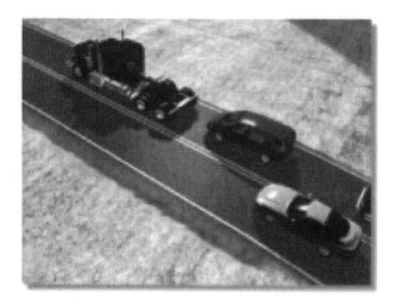

car behind you is trying to push you forward.

Summary

The cells in the body are designed to run at -20 to -25 millivolts. To heal by making new cells, we must achieve -50 millivolts. We get chronically sick when voltage drops to below -20 millivolts.

When voltage drops to below -20 millivolts, we get chronic pain. In addition, oxygen levels drop since they are controlled by the voltage level. When oxygen levels drop, metabolism changes to where we only get 2 molecules of ATP instead of 38 molecules per unit of fat processed. Cells struggle to function when they are getting "two miles to the gallon". In addition, the trillion or so "bugs" that are always in our bodies wake up when oxygen levels drop. They begin to "have lunch" by putting out enzymes that dissolve our cells. These enzymes enter our blood and damage cells throughout the body.

Thus chronic disease is always defined by low voltage.

To measure our voltages, we can easily use the acupuncture meridians. These are simply the fascial "wires" that connect every cell in the body. We use the Assess Mode of the Tennant BioModulator to measure each point called the Tennant BioTerminals. That gives us the voltage of the attached organs. We can also measure the Tesla Circuits that monitor the voltages in each circuit.

Now that we know the voltages in each organ, we can support the low ones by using the Tennant BioModulator. We must, however, begin the search for why the voltage was low enough to allow the person to get sick in the first place. That is the subject of the remainder of the book.

3 BioModulator

FDA Statement

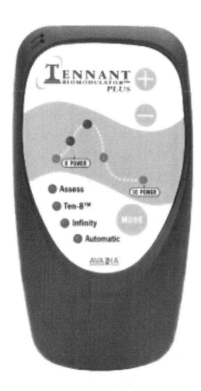

The Tennant Biomodulator®[1] and certain accessory electrodes are FDA listed by its distributor or manufacturer in these categories:
21 CFR 882.5890 – Neurology transcutaneous electrical nerve stimulator for pain relief
21 CFR 882.5050 – Neurology biofeedback device

Indications for use:
•Symptomatic relief and management of chronic,
•intractable pain.
- Adjunctive treatment in the management of post-traumatic surgical and post-traumatic pain
- Relaxation training and muscle relaxation

For more information, see www.senergy.us

Care of the BioModulator:
1. Don't turn on if below freezing.
2. Clean with alcohol sponge and wipe gently.
3. Clean electrode with alcohol sponge between people.

4. Do not drop!!!

5. Device can be damaged to the point of non-function if dropped on hard surface.

6. Device will be damaged beyond repair if dropped in water or liquids are spilled inside.

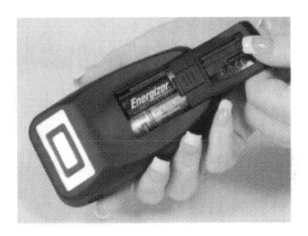

7. Device uses 2 AA alkaline batteries.

8. When ON/OFF switch is in the ON position, device is still powered and battery life is being used.

9. Initial batteries included with the device have a clear plastic covering. Remove it before placing the batteries in the battery compartment.

10. Battery compartment cover slides on/off the device.

11. Do NOT force battery cover or push it down. This can cause breakage of cover clips – non-warranty item.

The ON/OFF switch is on the side of the unit. There is an accessory port on the other side of the unit.

The power is adjusted with the plus and minus buttons.

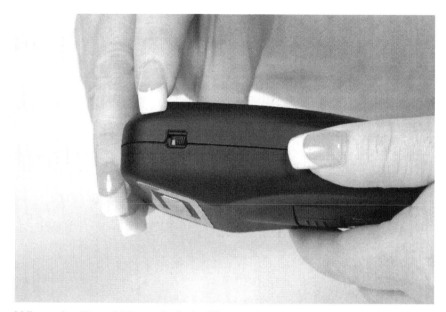

When in Ten-8™ or Infinity™ modes, the illuminated LEDs show the power settings, and are NOT reflecting the assessed value as is the case in the Assess or Automatic mode.

Turn the device on. Press and hold the (+) button. Watch the LEDs illuminate progressively up the curve (left to right) as the power level increases.

At the bottom range of each diode, the LED flashes. At the upper end of the range, the LED is solid. As the power increases, the next LED will begin to flash.

By convention we say that:
1. Below-threshold level of energy does not give subjective sensation.
2. Threshold level is sensed as slight vibration. This is the most commonly used setting

3. Above-threshold level is sensed as comfortable tingling sensation.
4. Supra-threshold level is sensed as uncomfortable.

It is better to use too little power than too much. The device operates in volts – cells in millivolts. They will shut down if you use too much power. Let children control the power themselves.

Modes:

Assess – Acts as your "voltmeter" to measure musculoskeletal problems or organ voltage.

Ten-8™ – Use for pain and musculoskeletal issues.

Infinity™ Use for everything else or alternate with Ten-8™.

Automatic (or Automatic Infinity™) The software measures the voltage and then treats with Infinity for one minute.

To use the BioModulator, you must adjust the power for the thickness of skin you wish to measure. Then put it into Assess Mode. Press firmly over the area in question. The lights will tell you the voltage according to the image above. Now measure the BioTerminals described in the chapter of Voltage.

Remember that chronic diseases are characterized by low voltage. Voltages drop before blood tests become abnormal. Blood tests become abnormal before you have symptoms. Wherever you find low voltages, the organs served by those BioTerminals will be struggling now or in the future.

Setting Power
According to Skin Thickness

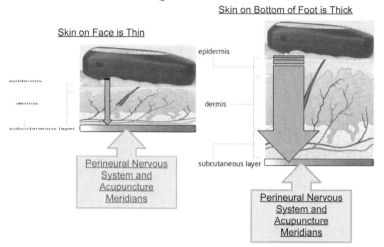

Look at the chart.. It will confirm for you which BioTerminal is associated with various illnesses. It is generally intuitive. For example, eye problems will have low voltage in the skull BioTerminal. Heart problems will have low voltage in the chest BioTerminal. Bladder problems will have low voltage in the Pelvic BioTerminal, etc.

BioTransducer

When we are using the BioModulator on the skin, we are primarily treating via the acupuncture meridians or the perineural nervous system. For most things, this works well. However, there is a more efficient way to get electrons into deep or swollen areas. It is with the use of an attachment to the BioModulator called the BioTransducer.

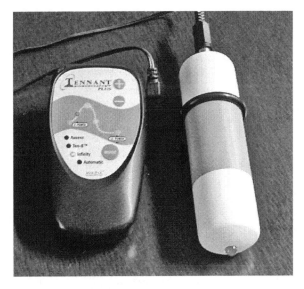

If I put an electrode on each side of my door, electrons will not flow from one to the other because the door is an insulator. If I shine a light on the door, it won't penetrate either. However, if I place a magnet on each side of the door, they will hold onto each other as their magnetic fields interact.

Remember that tissue with low voltage always creates a magnetic field. We call those "stickies" as we move the BioModulator over them.

The BioTransducer creates a magnetic field. We modulate the BioModulator frequencies onto the BioTransducer's magnetic field. By doing so, we are able to send the frequencies through solid material like the skull and brain, other bones, and into deep organs like the heart and liver. The BioTransducer thus gives us a more efficient way to get the electrons into deep organs like the brain.

When we move the BioTransducer over an area, when we contact the magnetic field of low voltage, we will feel it stick just the same way we feel a sticky on the skin. When the

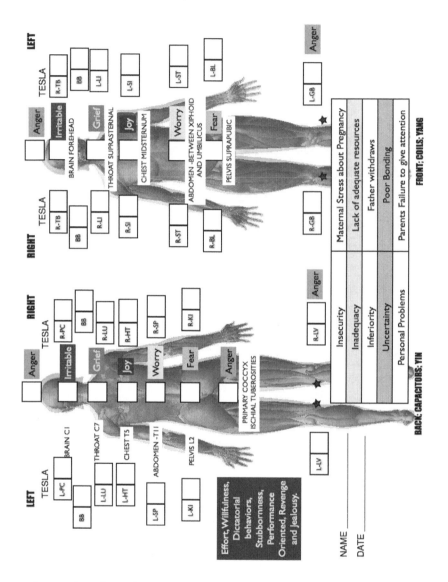

voltage in the deep organ is corrected, the sticky spot disappears and we know that we have corrected that area.

The trick to learning how to use the BioTransducer is to stop thinking about what you are doing and close out as many external sensory inputs as you can. Dim the lights, turn off the music, stop talking, get relaxed, and just let you hand take the BioTransducer wherever it seems to want to do. Soon you will feel the sticky. With practice, you will soon do it without thinking about it.

It's a little like learning to ride a bicycle. When we first climb on, we are tense and our movements are jerky. We can never really ride until we relax. After we do that, our movements become automatic and we stop thinking about how to ride. So it is with the BioTransducer. You will find the stickies quickly when you stop thinking about where they are.

Using the BioModulator

Now let's look at some examples of how one can use the BioModulator to help identify and confirm various illnesses.

A woman had a tooth extracted. The socket became infected and she was placed on antibiotics. Still the area would not heal. She was given different antibiotics, both orally and intravenously. Still the area would not heal. Repeat surgery to remove the infected bone still did not allow the area to heal.

Now let's look at her voltages. What you can see is that most of her voltages are low since they should all be 20 to 25 millivolts. Almost all of the voltages to the solid organs are low-voltage. You will recall that the solid organs are attached to the BioTerminals on the back. Also, all but two of the BioTerminals on the front (hollow organs) are low as well.

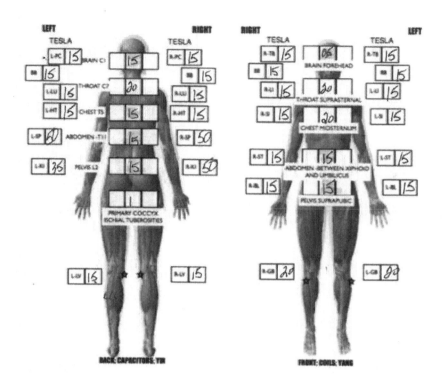

When the average of these numbers is less than 20, we realized that the patient has low total body voltage. Low total body voltage is hypothyroidism until proven otherwise. Remember that the blood tests are usually misleading.

I looked at her hypothyroidism questionnaire. This questionnaire asks the person to indicate which symptoms of hypothyroidism are present and how severe they are. The maximum score possible is 42. This patient rated 42. In addition, her physical exam was characteristic of hypothyroidism.

Now look at the numbers from the corresponding Tesla circuits. You will see that almost all of these are low. When these are low, you almost always find that the adrenals are fatigued. Her adrenal questionnaire scored 48/51, confirming that she has adrenal fatigue.

Now focus on the BioTerminals for the skull. The posterior one is 15 and the anterior one is 5. Thus the voltage to all the organs/structures in the skull is inadequate for healing. Do you remember what voltage it takes to heal? You're right! It's -50 millivolts. Now we know exactly why this person can't heal the infection in her jaw. She simply doesn't have the voltage to do it.

The solution now is easy. Use the BioModulator to insert electrons into the skull BioTerminals. In addition we can use the BioTransducer to use magnetic fields to get the electrons down into the center of the jaw (the acupuncture meridians will take them to the periosteum of the jaw but it will be more difficult for them to get into the center of the infection without the BioTransducer).

While we are actively providing the electrons necessary to heal the jaw, we must also deal with the rest of the body. It will give us the support system necessary to heal. We start correcting the hypothyroidism and the adrenal fatigue with desiccated hormones, iodine, vitamins, minerals, etc. needed to get them functioning as we have discussed in other chapters.

Remember that the immune system needs voltage, iodine, and ozone to kill bugs. We will aggressively start restoring her deficiency of iodine so her "iodine shield" can be restored to prevent new infections.

Remember that sodium chlorite works the same way as the white blood cells kill bugs---oxidation. So we would also use a short burst of sodium chlorite to help kill the infections. She will be full of L-forms because of all the antibiotics she has taken. Remember that sodium chlorite is an electron stealer, so we would not want to use it more than a week or two to attempt to get ahead of the infection. We would use the BioModulator and BioTransducer as much as possible to restore the electrons consumed by the sodium chlorite.

Remember also that low voltage causes low oxygen. We would use hyperbaric oxygen if that were available.

This person perfectly demonstrates what happens when voltage drops. First she became hypothyroid. Fluoride would have had a lot to do with this---also soy consumption and consuming things that act like estrogen. This dropped her voltage so it was hard for her to get her work done. However, her adrenals kept pushing to get her through the day. After a while, they gave up as well.

Low voltage caused by the hypothyroidism allowed the following things to happen:
    Chronic pain
    Decreased oxygen
    Decreased production of ATP
    Infections including L-forms that never respond to antibiotics

Addition of antibiotics made even more L-forms. They don't respond to anything except changing the voltage of the environment. (Sodium chlorite works via voltage change, not biochemically like antibiotics).

Let's look at another person. This man worked with gasoline and diesel and grease most of his life. He developed cancer of his left kidney. The left kidney was removed but no chemotherapy or radiation was used. Nine years later, he was found to have tumors in his pancreas, left hip, and lungs. He chose not to have chemotherapy or radiation but instead changed his diet and did nutritional things to improve his immune system. He also did a lot of detoxification. Two years later, the lung tumors are gone, the tumor in the left hip is smaller, and the tumor in the pancreas has not

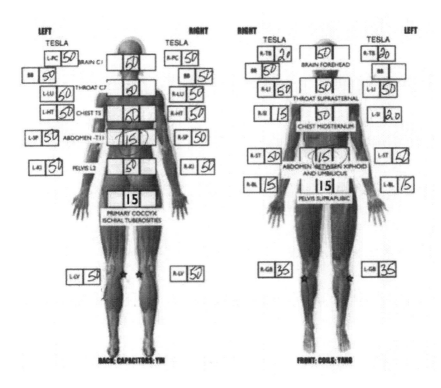

changed in size.

Look at his voltages. Most of his body is running at 50 millivolts. His body is actively in a healing mode. Fortunately for him, he is not hypothyroid or hypo-adrenal. Otherwise, he could not mount this healing effort.

Note, however, that his voltage is low in the Abdominal BioTerminal. It is 15 both back and front. This of course corresponds with the pancreas. Thus he has not been able to resolve this tumor and is at risk of it growing as long as the voltages are low.

Look at the Pelvic numbers. The voltage is low in the pelvis placing this area at risk. It also explains why he has a tumor in the hip.

This emphasizes the importance of measuring and knowing the voltage numbers. He is feeling great. The only way he knows that he is at significant risk for the tumors growing again is that the voltages are low. Tumors can't grow if the oxygen levels are normal, and oxygen levels are controlled by voltage. He must get the voltages up in the Abdominal and Pelvic BioTerminals. I suggested that he wear the BioModulator 24 hours per day with patches attached to those BioTerminals.

When only one or a few BioTerminals have low voltage, you should suspect a dental infection in the same circuit or in a Tesla that controls that BioTerminal. For example, with low Abdominal BioTerminals, the back Tesla is the Spleen circuit and the front Tesla is the Stomach. Look for infected teeth in those circuits using this chart. That would be teeth 2,

3,14,15, 20, 21, 28, or 29.   Measure any metal in these
teeth with a voltmeter as I described in the dental chapter. If
there is a root canal in one of these teeth, you know why the
voltage dropped. It must be removed or you will never get
the voltages back to normal.

The Pelvic BioTerminal is controlled by the Kidney Tesla on
the back and the Bladder Tesla on the front.   Look for
problems in teeth number 7, 8, 9, 10, 23, 24, 25, or 26 to
help explain why this BioTerminal is low. Also remember that
if you have a root canal, it will infect the bone and then infect
the bone of its next-door neighbors.   For example, a root
canal in tooth 27 (liver, gall bladder) could take out the
kidney, bladder circuit of tooth 26.

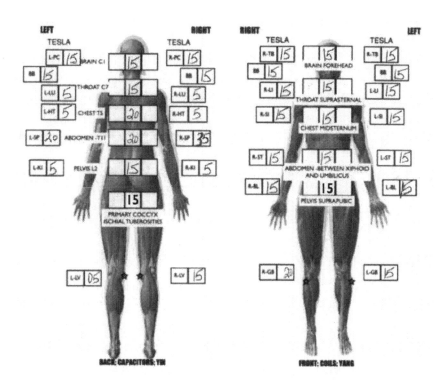

This next person is a teenage boy. He developed Crohn's Disease. *Crohn's disease (also known as granulomatous, and colitis) is an inflammatory disease of the intestines that may affect any part of the gastrointestinal tract from mouth to anus, causing a wide variety of symptoms. It primarily causes abdominal pain, diarrhea (which may be bloody), vomiting, or weight loss, but may also cause complications outside of the gastrointestinal tract such as skin rashes, arthritis, inflammation of the eye, tiredness, and lack of concentration.*

Crohn's disease is thought to be an autoimmune disease, in which the body's immune system attacks the gastrointestinal tract, causing inflammation; it is classified as a type of inflammatory bowel disease. Wikipedia

In addition to the Crohn's Disease, this boy has uveitis, an inflammation of the eyes.   It is also thought to be an autoimmune disease although uveitis has been thought by many over the years to be associated with infections, particularly fungal infections.

He recently was hospitalized for dehydration from diarrhea. While in the hospital, he contracted Clostridium difficile. We discussed this terrible infection in the chapter on infections.

He has been given large doses of antibiotics.   He has developed an anal fistula.

Look at his voltages.   Remember that for children or athletes, normal voltage is minus 30-35 millivolts.   His readings average 14.6 millivolts. Thus his total body voltage is half what it should be! Now you understand why he isn't getting well.

The primary things that lower total body voltage are hypothyroidism, narcotic drug use, epilepsy drugs, and losing sleep when you have little reserve.

This boy's hypothyroidism questionnaire is 17/42. This makes hypothyroidism most likely. The low numbers in his Tesla circuits support his adrenals being worn out as well. With low voltages and low adrenal function, his immune system cannot deal with infections. The heavy use of antibiotics will have created large numbers of L-forms that are resistant to antibiotics.

As voltage drops more and more, the end result is fungal forms that are cell-wall deficient. These are the most pathological forms of infections. They do not respond to antibiotics, cannot be cultured, and are only seen with a phase contrast or darkfield microscope. They can most easily be seen with a Grayfield microscope.

It is of some interest that uveitis has been associated with fungus for over 50 years, but it has always been difficult to prove because the fungus can rarely be cultured!

This boy's diet is primarily canned food. It is full of soy and plastic Trans fats. Soy shuts down the entire endocrine system. Soybeans are high in phytic acid, present in the bran or hulls of all seeds. It's a substance that can block the uptake of essential minerals (calcium, magnesium, copper, iron and especially zinc) in the intestinal tract.

Zinc is called the intelligence mineral because it is needed for optimal development and functioning of the brain and nervous system. It plays a role in protein synthesis and collagen formation; it is involved in the blood-sugar control mechanism and thus protects against diabetes; it is needed for a healthy reproductive system.

Zinc is a key component in numerous vital enzymes and plays a role in the immune system.

Phytates found in soy products interfere with zinc absorption more completely than with other minerals.

Zinc deficiency can cause a "spacey" feeling that some vegetarians may mistake for the "high" of spiritual enlightenment.

One of the problems with canned food is the presence of Trans fats and Canola oil. Canola oil stunts the growth of infants. It is not suitable for human consumption. However, the discussion of Canola is beyond the scope of this book. Trans fats will not make good cell membranes. Cells made with Trans fats cannot hold a charge and cause the voltage to be low. You see that regularly in brain-injured people. The brain replaces itself in 8 months. About six months after a brain injured person is put on canned food containing high amounts of Trans fats, the nervous system stops getting better. A brain made of plastic just doesn't work!

The same is true when other people are put on canned food as their primary diet. Look at this boy's voltage. Part of the low voltage is due to cell membranes made from plastic Trans fats.

Fats of any kind (except coconut oil) cannot be absorbed without bile, so one needs to pay attention to whether the liver is capable of making bile. A liver running on half-normal voltage will not be able to do so. Thus one must supplement bile and digestive enzymes until the voltage normalizes.

I would recommend that this boy wear the BioModulator 24 hours a day while we are changing his diet, and correcting his thyroid function and adrenals, stomach acid, etc.

Macular Degeneration

Macular degeneration is becoming an increasing problem as people age. Ophthalmologists believe they have two options to treat it. If bleeding isn't present, it's treated with vitamins. If bleeding is present, the eye is injected with drugs intended to shut down blood vessels. Neither work very well. The reason is, of course, that's it's all about the voltage in the eye.

What BioTerminal would provide the voltage to the eye? The skull or head BioTerminal of course. It will always be low in people with macular degeneration.

Note in the person with macular degeneration that the posterior Head BioTerminal has 15 millivolts and the anterior reads 05 millivolts. The Tesla circuits that monitor the Head BioTerminals are the Triple Burner and the Pericardium. Note that the Triple Burner Teslas are reading 05.

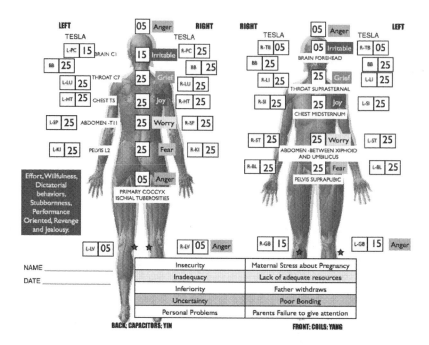

The Head gets voltage delivered from the Primary Cable. The Primary Cable is controlled by the Liver and Gall Bladder Teslas.   Thus they also have an effect on the structures of the head including the eye. Note that the Liver Teslas are at 05 at the coccyx and at the top of the head (GV-20).   Now we know why the person has macular degeneration. The voltage supply is diminished.

Look at the dental chart.   This person has a root canal in tooth #6. He has a crown on tooth #22 that measures 180 millivolts with a voltmeter (means there is infection under the crown). This person has low voltage in the eyes because of infection in the teeth that are on the same circuits.

Acumeridian Tooth-Organ Relationships [with Autonomic Neuropeptide Emotion correlations] -- from various sources. Dr. Ralph Wilson, ND

Tooth	Organ	Emotions
1	Heart, Small Int., Circulation/Sex, Endocrine	Loneliness; Acute Grief; Humiliated; Trapped; Imitative; Greed; Not lovable
2	Pancreas, Stomach	Anxiety; Overcritical; Broken Power; Hate; Low self-worth; Obsessed
3	Pancreas, Stomach	Anxiety; Overcritical; Broken Power; Hate; Low self-worth; Obsessed
4	Lung, Large Intestine	Chronic Grief; Controlling, Feeling trapped; Dogmatic; Upright
5	Lung, Large Intestine	Chronic Grief; Controlling, Feeling trapped; Dogmatic; Upright
6	Liver, Gallbladder	Anger; Resentment; Frustration; Blaming; Inescapable; have action; Manipulative
7	Kidney, Bladder	Fear, Shame; Guilt; Broken will; Shyness, Helpless; Deep exhaustion
8	Kidney, Bladder	Fear, Shame; Guilt; Broken will; Shyness, Helpless; Deep exhaustion
9	Kidney, Bladder	Fear, Shame; Guilt; Broken will; Shyness, Helpless; Deep exhaustion
10	Kidney, Bladder	Fear, Shame; Guilt; Broken will; Shyness, Helpless; Deep exhaustion
11	Liver, Gallbladder	Anger; Resentment; Frustration; Blaming; Inescapable; have action; Manipulative
12	Lung, Large Intestine	Chronic Grief; Controlling, Feeling trapped; Dogmatic; Upright
13	Lung, Large Intestine	Chronic Grief; Controlling, Feeling trapped; Dogmatic; Upright
14	Stomach, Spleen	Anxiety; Self-Punishment; Broken Power; Hate; Low self-worth; Obsessed
15	Stomach, Spleen	Anxiety; Self-Punishment; Broken Power; Hate; Low self-worth; Obsessed
16	Heart, Small Int., Circulation/Sex, Endocrine	Loneliness; Acute Grief; Humiliated; Trapped; Imitative; Greed; Not lovable

The person was sent to the dentist to pull the root canal tooth including removing any infection in the associated bone. The crown on #22 must be removed and the decay and any mercury under it must be removed and the crown replaced.

108

The BioModulator is used to restore voltage to the Head BioTerminals. In addition, the BioTransducer is used to place voltage directly on the retina.

Our study of dry macular degeneration showed that if the vision is better than 20/70, we got them all back to 20/20 or 20/25. If there was enough scarring that the vision was worse than 20/70, we did not get back to the vision necessary to read easily (20/50) but the vision did not get worse over the next two years.

Summary

I have attempted to give only a few examples of the usefulness of the BioModulator and a voltmeter in determining the underlying cause of illness = low voltage. You can expand the examples to almost any illness. The location of the illness usually tells you the BioTerminal that will have low voltage. You will quickly learn which Tesla circuits monitors each BioTerminal.

There are a couple of non-intuitive connections for the BioTerminal and Tesla circuits. The large intestine is served partly by the Neck BioTerminal because of the way it is formed embryonically. Other parts are served by the Abdomen and the Pelvic BioTerminals. In addition, the breast is served by the Abdomen BioTerminal and the Stomach Tesla.

There are a few special considerations that are beyond the scope of this handbook. However, the purpose of this handbook is to give one the basic concepts. Training is available for those wishing to learn the nuances.

4 Dental Toxins

If you have a computer nearby, I would like you to stop reading and watch the following videos:

Smoking Teeth at http://www.youtube.com/watch?v=9ylnQ-T7oiA

How Mercury Causes Brain Neuron Damage at http://www.youtube.com/watch?v=XU8nSn5Ezd8&feature=related

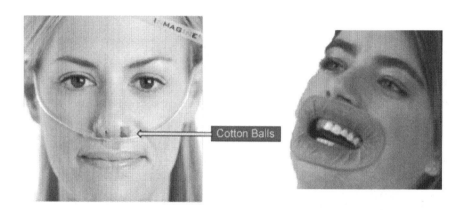

Cotton Balls

Obviously, if you have mercury fillings in your mouth, you must get them SAFELY removed. This means that your dentist needs to give you an auxiliary air supply so you won't breath the mercury vapors coming out of your mouth as the dentist drills out the mercury. You also need a dental rubber dam. This is a piece of rubber. The dentist pokes the tooth in question through the rubber sheet. It then captures the pieces of mercury that fall into your mouth so you don't swallow them. If you don't follow these precautions, the mercury will be moved from your mouth to your brain!

You must realize that every tooth is wired into an acupuncture meridian. Whatever happens to that tooth happens to the meridian. However, the meridians are like

Loneliness, Acute Grief, Humiliated, Trapped, Inhibited, Greed, Not lovable	Anxiety, Self-Punishment, Broken Power, Hate, Low self-worth, Obsessed	Chronic Grief, Overcritical, Sadness, Controlling, Feeling trapped, Dogmatic, Compulsive, Uptight	Anger, Resentment, Frustration, Blaming, Incapable to take action, Manipulative	Fear, Shame, Guilt, Broken will, Shyness, Helpless, Deep exhaustion
Duodenum, Middle Ear, Shoulder, Elbow, CNS	Sinus: Maxillary, Oropharynx, Larynx	Sinus: Paranasal and Ethmoid, Bronchus, Nose	Sinus: Sphenoid, Palatine Tonsil, Hip, Eye, Knee	Sinus: Frontal, Pharyngeal Tonsil, Genito-Urinary System
Heart, Small Int., Circulation/Sex, Endocrine	**Pancreas Stomach**	**Lung Large Intestine**	**Liver Gallbladder**	**Kidney Bladder**

1	2	3	4	5	6	7	8

32	31	30	29	28	27	26	25

Heart, Small Int., Circulation/Sex, Endocrine	**Lung Large Intestine**	**Pancreas Stomach**	**Liver Gallbladder**	**Kidney Bladder**
Shoulder, Elbow, Ileum, Middle Ear, Peripheral Nerves	Sinus: Paranasal and Ethmoid, Bronchus, Nose	Sinus: Maxillary, Larynx, Lymph, Oropharynx, Breast, Knee	Sinus: Sphenoid, Palatine Tonsil, Hip, Eye, Knee	Sinus: Frontal, Ear, Pharyngeal Tonsil, Genito-Urinary System
Loneliness, Acute Grief, Humiliated, Trapped, Inhibited, Greed, Not lovable	Chronic Grief, Overcritical, Sadness, Controlling, Feeling trapped, Dogmatic, Compulsive, Uptight	Anxiety, Self-Punishment, Broken Power, Hate, Low self-worth, Obsessed	Anger, Resentment, Frustration, Blaming, Incapable to take action, Manipulative	Fear, Shame, Guilt, Broken will, Shyness, Helpless, Deep exhaustion

Acumeridian Tooth-Organ Relationships [with Autonomic/Neurop

Fear, Shame, Guilt, Broken will, Shyness, Helpless, Deep exhaustion	Anger, Resentment Frustration, Blaming, Incapable to take action, Manipulative	Chronic Grief, Overcritical, Sadness, Controlling, Feeling trapped, Dogmatic, Compulsive, Uptight	Anxiety, Self-Punishment, Broken Power, Hate, Low self-worth, Obsessed	Loneliness, Acute Grief, Humiliated, Trapped, Inhibited, Greed, Not lovable
Sinus: Frontal Pharyngeal Tonsil Genito-Urinary System	Sinus: Sphenoid Palatine Tonsil Hip, Eye, Knee	Sinus: Paranasal and Ethmoid, Bronchus, Nose	Sinus: Maxillary Oropharynx Larynx	Ileum, Jejunum Middle Ear, Shoulder Elbow, CNS
Kidney Bladder	**Liver Gallbladder**	**Lung Large Intestine**	**Stomach Spleen**	**Heart, Small Int., Circulation/Sex, Endocrine**

9	10	11	12	13	14	15	16
24	23	22	21	20	19	18	17

Kidney Bladder	**Liver Gallbladder**	**Spleen Stomach**	**Lung Large Intestine**	**Heart, Small Int., Circulation/Sex, Endocrine**
Sinus: Frontal Ear, Pharyngeal Tonsil Genito-Urinary System	Sinus: Sphenoid Palatine Tonsil Hip, Eye Knee	Sinus: Maxillary Larynx, Lymph, Oropharynx Breast Knee	Sinus: Paranasal and Ethmoid, Bronchus, Nose	Shoulder, Elbow Ileum, Jejunum, Middle Ear Peripheral Nerves
Fear, Shame, Guilt, Broken will, Shyness, Helpless, Deep exhaustion	Anger, Resentment Frustration, Blaming, Incapable to take action, Manipulative	Anxiety, Self-Punishment, Broken Power, Hate, Low self-worth, Obsessed	Chronic Grief, Overcritical, Sadness, Controlling, Feeling trapped, Dogmatic, Compulsive, Uptight	Loneliness, Acute Grief, Humiliated, Trapped, Inhibited, Greed, Not lovable

eptide Emotion correlations] -- from various sources Dr. Ralph Wilson, N.D.

Christmas lights with multiple bulbs on them. Meridians are wires with multiple organs including a tooth on the same circuit. If you remove a light bulb, the circuit is still there. If you remove your gall bladder, your gall bladder circuit is still present.

As you can see from the following graphic, teeth are wired into the circuits. Notice for example, the breast is

Meridians by System			
Armpit	Heart		
Adrenals	Kidney		
Body Fluids	Bladder		
Brain	Heart	Spleen/Pancreas	Bladder
Breast	Stomach		
Cardiovascular	Pericardium		
Depression	Lung	Sanjaio	Pericardium
Ear	Small Intestine	Kidney	Gall Bladder
Emotions	Gall Bladder		
Endocrine	Spleen/Pancreas	Gall Bladder	Kidneys (adrenals)
Eye	Sanjaio	Liver	Bladder
Eyelid (Upper)	Stomach		
Fatigue	Heart	Sanjaio	
Gonads	Liver		
Head	Pericardium	Gall Bladder	
Large Intestine	Lung	Small Intestine	
Lips	Stomach		
Lung	Pericardium		
Lymph	Sanjaio		
Mouth	Stomach		
Mucous Membranes	Bladder		
Neck	Small Intestine		
Nervous System	Kidney		
Nose	Lung	Large Intestine	Bladder
Parasympathetic	Pericardium		
Ribs	Spleen/Pancreas	Liver	
Shoulder	Large Intestine	Lung	Stomach	Spleen/Pancreas
Skin	Lung	Large Intestine	Pericardium	Heart
Stomach	Spleen/Pancreas		
Sympathetic	Sanjaio		
Tongue	Heart		
Tooth	Large Intestine		

wired into the stomach circuit. Another way of thinking about it is that the breast gets its voltage from the same wire or circuit as the stomach does. That means that if you have an infection in an upper molar (stomach meridian), that infection will affect the breast on that side as well as the stomach.

The BioTerminals help you know the primary source of voltage for each circuit.

In addition many organs have more than one wire that takes voltage to it.

Organs on Meridians					
Lung	Nose	Skin	Large Intestine	Shoulder and back	Depression
Pericardium	Cardiovascular	Parasympathetic	Neurochemical	Lung	Head
Heart	Brain	Armpit	Tongue	Skin	Cardiovascular
Small Intestine	Ear	Neck	Large Intestine		
Sanjaio (Triple Heater)	Lymph	Eye	Sympathetic		
Large Intestine	Skin	Nose	Shoulder	Tooth	
Spleen/Pancreas	Brain	Stomach	Ribs	Endocrine	
Liver	Gonads	Ribs	Eye		
Kidney	Adrenals	Ear	Nervous system		
Bladder	Brain	Eye	Nose	Body fluids	Mucous Membranes
Gall Bladder	Head	Ear	Endocrine	Emotions	
Stomach	Breast	Mouth	Nose	Lips	Upper lid

In this chart, you see that the wire called the lung meridian also takes voltage to the nose, skin, large intestine, and shoulder. The wire called the stomach meridian takes voltage to the stomach, breast, mouth, nose, lips and upper lid.

In the previous chart, you will see that some organs have multiple wires supplying voltage to them. For example, the brain gets voltage from the heart, spleen/pancreas, and bladder circuits. The eye gets voltage from the triple burner (sanjiao), liver, and bladder circuits. If you study the BioTerminal circuits above, you will see that the primary BioTerminal for the eyes is in the center of the forehead. It is modulated by the Triple Burner circuit from the hand and receives voltage from the liver circuit that is attached to the top of the head.

Don't let all of this confuse you. If you want to keep it simple, just focus on the BioTerminals to provide voltage. However, when you are considering if a certain tooth is causing trouble with the organ you are interested in, look at the meridian charts above. See what wires are carrying voltage to the organs you are interested in. Then look to see if you have an infection in a tooth in one of those circuits. If so, you have the reason that the voltage dropped enough in that circuit to allow the person to get sick.

There is often a recurring pattern with teeth. You get a small cavity. The dentist removes about 1/3 of the tooth with undercuts so that mercury amalgam filling won't fall out. This weakens the tooth. Soon it fractures. The dentist then puts a crown on the tooth without removing the amalgam. Now you have an open wound in the tooth with mercury leaking into it. Decay happens but the dentist cannot detect it because x-rays won't penetrate the crown so the x-ray looks fine. Next comes pain. The dentist then recommends a root canal.

A root canal is performed by drilling a small hole into the biting surface of the tooth. An auger is then inserted into the root of the tooth and the artery and nerve are ripped out.

Everyone knows that dead tissue in the body always gets infected. That is why it is surprising that dentists purposefully leave dead teeth in the mouth. The dentists are the only physicians that purposely leave dead tissue in the body!

Most dentists are convinced that they can seal the tooth so that infection in the tooth is impossible. Unfortunately, that is wishful thinking. This study published in the root canal doctors' own journal shows the problem clearly. They took patients that were going to have wisdom teeth removed. They did a root canal on one tooth. Then three months later they removed both teeth. What you see is that the untreated

Nagaoka, et al. (1995). Bacterial invasion into dentinal tubules of human vital and non-vital teeth.
J. Endodon. 21: 70-73

Vital Tooth   **Non-vital Root Canal Tooth**

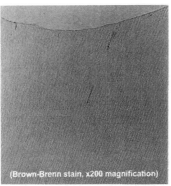
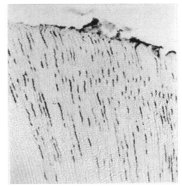

(Brown-Brenn stain, x200 magnification)

% Invaded Tubules: 1.1%   vs.   39.0%

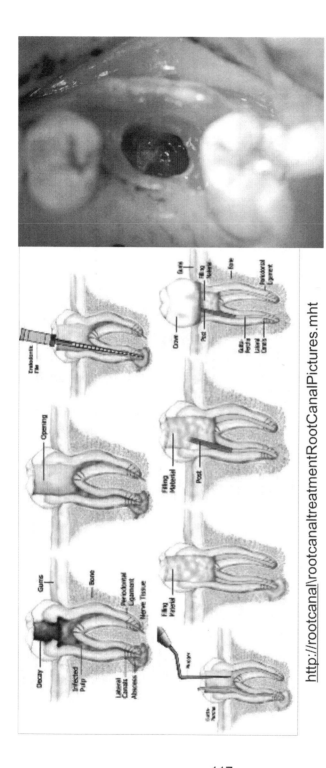

http://rootcanal\rootcanaltreatmentRootCanalPictures.mht

117

tooth had 1.1% of the tubules infected. However, the tooth that had the root canal performed three months earlier had infection in 39% of the tubules!

A study done at the University of Kentucky looked at the effects of root canal toxins on the immune system. When the teeth are infected with bacteria, they produce a toxin called thio-ethers. When the infection is caused by fungus, it

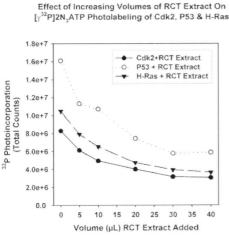

Effect of Increasing Volumes of RCT Extract On
$[\gamma^{32}P]2N_3ATP$ Photolabeling of Cdk2, P53 & H-Ras

File Name: 111402A.JNB

CDK2 is noted here with the solid line with black circles at the bottom. CDK2 with root canal extract showed 26% inhibition at 5 ul and 63% inhibition at 40 ul. So this one produced a pretty flat graph curve with the most inhibition in the first half of the test.

produces glio-toxins.

CDK2 is noted here with the solid line with black circles at the bottom. CDK2 with root canal extract showed 26% inhibition at 5 ul and 63% inhibition at 40 ul. Thus one root canal shuts down 63% of the immune system. Most of that is focused on the acupuncture meridian attached to that tooth.

Having poisonous mercury coming from your teeth is one problem. Another problem just as severe is having an

Adriaens et al., (1988). *J. Clin. Periodontol.*

59:493-503.∎

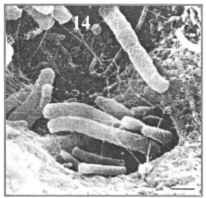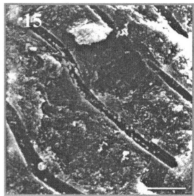

"Figure 14. Filamentous bacteria invading the dentinal tubules at their orifices in the bottom of a resorption lacuna."

"Figure 15. Longitudinally fractured dentinal tubules in the radicular dentin area corresponding to the exposed subgingival root surface. Bacteria are present in the dentinal tubules."

infected tooth. The teeth that are always infected are root canal teeth, but any cavity or infection under a crown releases the same toxins.

The following interview is from Dr. Joseph Mercola: www.mercola.com

Effective Non-Drug Non-Surgical Solutions for Chronic Illnesses
Dr. Joseph Mercola
1443 W. Schaumburg Rd.
Schaumburg, IL 60194-4065
'Phone 847-985-1777

ROOT CANALS POSE HEALTH THREAT - AN INTERVIEW WITH George Meinig, D.D.S.

Dr. Meinig brings a most curious perspective to an expose of latent dangers of root canal therapy - fifty years ago he was one of the founders of the American Association of

Endodontists (root canal specialists)! So he's filled his share of root canals. And when he wasn't filling canals himself, he was teaching the technique to dentists across the country at weekend seminars and clinics. About two years ago, having recently retired, he decided to read all 1174 pages of the detailed research of Dr. Weston Price, (D.D.S). Dr. Meinig was startled and shocked. Here was valid documentation of systemic illnesses resulting from latent infections lingering in filled roots. He has since written a book, "Root Canal Cover-Up EXPOSED - Many Illnesses Result", and is devoting himself to radio, TV, and personal appearances before groups in an attempt to blow the whistle and alert the public.

Dr. Mercola: Please explain what the problem is with root canal therapy.

George Meinig: First, let me note that my book is based on Dr. Weston Price's twenty-five years of careful, impeccable research. He led a 60-man team of researchers whose findings - suppressed until now rank right up there with the greatest medical discoveries of all time. This is not the usual medical story of a prolonged search for the difficult-to-find causative agent of some devastating disease. Rather, it's the story of how a "cast of millions" (of bacteria) become entrenched inside the structure of teeth and end up causing the largest number of diseases ever traced to a single source.

Dr. Mercola: What diseases? Can you give us some examples?

George Meinig: Yes, a high percentage of chronic degenerative diseases can originate from root filled teeth. The most frequent were heart and circulatory diseases and he found 16 different causative agents for these. The next most common diseases were those of the joints, arthritis and rheumatism. In third place - but almost tied for second - were diseases of the brain and nervous system. After that, any disease you can name might (and in some cases has) come from root filled teeth.

Let me tell you about the research itself. Dr. Price undertook his investigations in 1900. He continued until 1925, and published his work in two volumes in 1923. In 1915 the National Dental Association (which changed its name a few years later to The American Dental Association) was so impressed with his work that they appointed Dr. Price their first Research Director. His Advisory Board read like a Who's Who in medicine and dentistry for that era. They represented the fields of bacteriology, pathology, rheumatology, surgery, chemistry, and cardiology.
At one point in his writings Dr. Price made this observation: "Dr. Frank Billings (M.D.), probably more than any other American internist, is due credit for the early recognition of the importance of streptococcal focal infections in systemic involvements."

What's really unfortunate here is that very valuable information was covered up and totally buried some 70 years ago by a minority group of autocratic doctors who just didn't believe or couldn't grasp - the focal infection theory.
Dr. Mercola: What is the "focal infection" theory?
George Meinig: This states that germs from a central focal infection - such as teeth, teeth roots, inflamed gum tissues, or maybe tonsils - metastasize to hearts, eyes, lungs, kidneys, or other organs, glands and tissues, establishing new areas of the same infection. Hardly theory any more, this has been proven and demonstrated many times over. It's 100% accepted today. But it was revolutionary thinking during World War I days, and the early 1920's!
Today, both patients and physicians have been "brain washed" to think that infections are less serious because we now have antibiotics. Well, yes and no. In the case of root-filled teeth, the no longer-living tooth lacks a blood supply to its interior. So circulating antibiotics don't faze the bacteria living there because they can't get at them.

Dr. Mercola: You're assuming that ALL root-filled teeth harbor bacteria and/or other infective agents?

George Meinig: Yes. No matter what material or technique is used - and this is just as true today - the root filling shrinks minutely, perhaps microscopically. Further and this is key - the bulk of solid appearing teeth, called the dentin, actually consists of miles of tiny tubules. Microscopic organisms lurking in the maze of tubules simply migrate into the interior of the tooth and set up housekeeping. A filled root seems to be a favorite spot to start a new colony.

One of the things that makes this difficult to understand is that large, relatively harmless bacteria common to the mouth, change and adapt to new conditions. They shrink in size to fit the cramped quarters and even learn how to exist (and thrive!) on very little food. Those that need oxygen mutate and become able to get along without it. In the process of adaptation these formerly friendly "normal" organisms become pathogenic (capable of producing disease) and more virulent (stronger) and they produce much more potent toxins.
Today's bacteriologists are confirming the discoveries of the Price team of bacteriologists. Both isolated in root canals the same strains of streptococcus, staphylococcus and spirochetes.

Dr. Mercola: Is everyone who has ever had a root canal filled made ill by it?

George Meinig: No. We believe now that every root canal filling does leak and bacteria do invade the structure. But the variable factor is the strength of the person's immune system. Some healthy people are able to control the germs that escape from their teeth into other areas of the body. We think this happens because their immune system lymphocytes (white blood cells) and other disease fighters aren't constantly compromised by other ailments. In other words, they are able to prevent those new colonies from taking hold in other tissues throughout the body. But over time, most people with root filled teeth do seem to develop some kinds of systemic symptoms they didn't have before.

Dr. Mercola: It's really difficult to grasp that bacteria are imbedded deep in the structure of seemingly-hard, solid looking teeth.

George Meinig: I know. Physicians and dentists have that same problem, too. You really have to visualize the tooth structure - all of those microscopic tubules running through the dentin. In a healthy tooth, those tubules transport a fluid that carries nourishment to the inside. For perspective, if the tubules of a front single-root tooth, were stretched out on the ground they'd stretch for three miles!
A root filled tooth no longer has any fluid circulating through it, but the maze of tubules remains. The anaerobic bacteria that live there seem remarkably safe from antibiotics. The bacteria can migrate out into surrounding tissue where they can "hitch hike" to other locations in the body via the bloodstream. The new location can be any organ or gland or tissue, and the new colony will be the next focus of infection in a body plagued by recurrent or chronic infections.
All of the "building up" done to try to enhance the patient's ability to fight infections - to strengthen their immune system - is only a holding action. Many patients won't be well until the source of infection - the root canal tooth - is removed.

Dr. Mercola: I don't doubt what you're saying, but can you tell us more about how Dr. Price could be sure that arthritis or other systemic conditions and illnesses really originated in the teeth - or in a single tooth?

George Meinig: Yes. Many investigations start with the researcher just being curious about something - and then being scientifically careful enough to discover an answer, and then prove it's so, many times over. Dr. Price's first case is very well documented. He removed an infected tooth from a woman who suffered from severe arthritis. As soon as he finished with the patient, he implanted the tooth beneath the skin of a healthy rabbit. Within 48 hours the rabbit was crippled with arthritis!

Further, once the tooth was removed the patient's arthritis improved dramatically. This clearly suggested that the presence of the infected tooth was a causative agent for both that patient's and the rabbit's - arthritis.

[Editor's Note - Here's the story of that first patient from Dr. Meinig's book: "(Dr. Price) had a sense that, even when (root canal therapy) appeared successful, teeth containing root fillings remained infected. That thought kept prying on his mind, haunting him each time a patient consulted him for relief from some severe debilitating disease for which the medical profession could find no answer. Then one day while treating a woman who had been confined to a wheelchair for six years from severe arthritis, he recalled how bacterial cultures were taken from patients who were ill and then inoculated into animals in an effort to reproduce the disease and test the effectiveness of drugs on the disease.

With this thought in mind, although her (root filled) tooth looked fine, he advised this arthritic patient, to have it extracted. He told her he was going to find out what it was about this root filled tooth that was responsible for her suffering. "All dentists know that sometimes arthritis and other illnesses clear up if bad teeth are extracted. However, in this case, all of her teeth appeared in satisfactory condition and the one containing this root canal filling showed no evidence or symptoms of infection. Besides, it looked normal on x-ray pictures.

"Immediately after Dr. Price extracted the tooth he dismissed the patient and embedded her tooth under the skin of a rabbit. In two days the rabbit developed the same kind of crippling arthritis as the patient - and in ten days it died.

"..The patient made a successful recovery after the tooth's removal! She could then walk without a cane and could even do fine needlework again. That success led Dr. Price to advise other patients, afflicted with a wide variety of treatment defying illnesses, to have any root filled teeth out."]

In the years that followed, he repeated this procedure many hundreds of times. He later implanted only a portion of the tooth to see if that produced the same results. It did. He then dried the tooth, ground it into powder and injected a tiny bit into several rabbits. Same results, this time producing the same symptoms in multiple animals.

Dr. Price eventually grew cultures of the bacteria and injected them into the animals. Then he went a step further. He put the solution containing the bacteria through a filter small enough to catch the bacteria. So when he injected the resulting liquid it was free of any infecting bacteria. Did the test animals develop the illness? Yes. The only explanation was that the liquid had to contain toxins from the bacteria, and the toxins were also capable of causing disease.
Dr. Price became curious about which was the more potent infective agent, the bacteria or the toxin. He repeated that last experiment, injecting half the animals with the toxin-containing liquid and half of them with the bacteria from the filter. Both groups became ill, but the group injected with the toxins got sicker and died sooner than the bacteria injected animals.

Dr. Mercola: That's amazing. Did the rabbits always develop the same disease the patient had?

George Meinig: Mostly, yes. If the patient had heart disease the rabbit got heart disease. If the patient had kidney disease the rabbit got kidney disease, and so on. Only occasionally did a rabbit develop a different disease - and then the pathology would be quite similar, in a different location.

Dr. Mercola: If extraction proves necessary for anyone reading this, do you want to summarize what's special about the extraction technique?

George Meinig: Just pulling the tooth is not enough when removal proves necessary. Dr. Price found bacteria in the tissues and bone just adjacent to the tooth's root. So we now recommend slow-speed drilling with a burr, to remove one millimeter of the entire bony socket. The purpose is to remove the periodontal ligament (which is always infected with toxins produced by streptococcus bacteria living in the dentin tubules) and the first millimeter of bone that lines the socket (which is usually infected).

There's a whole protocol involved, including irrigating with sterile saline to assure removal of the contaminated bone chips, and treating the socket to stimulate and encourage infection-free healing. I describe the procedure in detail, step by step, in my book [pages 185 and 186].

Dr. Mercola: Perhaps we should back up and talk about oral health - to PREVENT needing an extraction. Caries or inflamed gums seem much more common than root canals. Do they pose any threat?

George Meinig: Yes, they absolutely do. But let me point out that we can't talk about oral health apart from total health. The problem is that patients and dentists alike haven't come around to seeing that dental caries reflect systemic - meaning "whole body" - illness. Dentists have learned to restore teeth so expertly that both they and their patients have come to regard tooth decay as a trivial matter. It isn't. Small cavities too often become big cavities. Big cavities too often lead to further destruction and the eventual need for root canal treatment.

Dr. Mercola: Then talk to us about prevention.

George Meinig: The only scientific way to prevent tooth decay is through diet and nutrition. Dr. Ralph Steinman did some outstanding, landmark research at Loma Linda University. He injected a glucose solution into mice - into their bodies, so the glucose didn't even touch their teeth. Then he observed the teeth for any changes. What he found was truly astonishing. The glucose reversed the normal flow of fluid in the dentin tubules, resulting in all of the test animals developing severe tooth decay! Dr. Steinman demonstrated dramatically what I said a minute ago: Dental caries reflect systemic illness.

Let's take a closer look to see how this might happen. Once a tooth gets infected and the cavity gets into the nerve and blood vessels, bacteria find their way into those tiny tubules of the dentin. Then no matter what we do by way of treatment, we're never going to completely eradicate the bacteria hiding in the miles of tubules. In time the bacteria can migrate through lateral canals into the surrounding bony socket that supports the tooth. Now the host not only has a cavity in a tooth, plus an underlying infection of supporting tissue to deal with, but the bacteria also exude potent systemic toxins. These toxins circulate throughout the body triggering activity by the immune system - and probably causing the host to feel less well. This host response can vary from just dragging around and feeling less energetic, to overt illness - of almost any kind. Certainly, such a person will be more vulnerable to whatever "bugs" are going around, because his/her body is already under constant challenge and the immune system continues to be "turned on" by either the infective agent or its toxins - or both.
Dr. Mercola: What a fascinating concept. Can you tell us more about the protective nutrition you mentioned?

George Meinig: Yes. Dr. Price traveled all over the world doing his research on primitive peoples who still lived in their native ways. He found fourteen cultural pockets scattered all over the globe where the natives had no access to "civilization" - and ate no refined foods.

Dr. Price studied their diets carefully. He found they varied greatly, but the one thing they had in common was that they ate whole, unrefined foods. With absolutely no access to tooth brushes, floss, fluoridated water or tooth paste, the primitive peoples studied were almost 100% free of tooth decay. Further - and not unrelated - they were also almost 100% free of all the degenerative diseases we suffer - problems with the heart, lungs, kidneys, liver, joints, skin (allergies), and the whole gamut of illnesses that plague Mankind. No one food proved to be magic as a preventive food. I believe we can thrive best by eating a wide variety of whole foods.

Dr. Mercola: Amazing. So by "diet and nutrition" for oral (and total) health you meant eating a pretty basic diet of whole foods?

George Meinig: Exactly. And no sugar or white flour. These are (and always have been) the first culprits. Tragically, when the primitives were introduced to sugar and white flour their superior level of health deteriorated rapidly. This has been demonstrated time and again. During the last sixty or more years we have added in increasing amounts, highly refined and fabricated cereals and boxed mixes of all kinds, soft drinks, refined vegetable oils and a whole host of other foodless "foods". It is also during those same years that we as a nation have installed more and more root canal fillings - and degenerative diseases have become rampant. I believe - and Dr. Price certainly proved to my satisfaction - that these simultaneous factors are NOT coincidences.

Dr. Mercola: I certainly understand what you are saying. But I'm still a little shocked to talk with a dentist who doesn't stress oral hygiene.

George Meinig: Well, I'm not against oral hygiene. Of course, hygiene practices are preventive, and help minimize the destructive effect of our "civilized", refined diet. But the real issue is still diet. The natives Dr. Price tracked down and studied weren't free of cavities, inflamed gums, and degenerative diseases because they had better tooth brushes!

Root Canals and Infected Bone

It's so easy to lose sight of the significance of what Dr. Price discovered. We tend to sweep it under the rug - we'd actually prefer to hear that if we would just brush better, longer, or more often, we too could be free of dental problems.
Certainly, part of the purpose of my book is to stimulate dental research into finding a way to sterilize dentin tubules. Only then can dentists really learn to save teeth for a lifetime. But the bottom line remains: A primitive diet of whole unrefined foods is the only thing that has been found to actually prevent both tooth decay and degenerative diseases.

One of the problems with root canals is that they often spread their infection into the surrounding bone. This is a huge problem since infections in bone are so hard to cure. They are often called "cavitations". Unfortunately these infections cannot be seen with standard dental x-rays. One can only see them with digital x-rays or 64-slice CAT scans."

The hole in the photo is where a root canal has been removed. You can see the blackened infected bone that surrounded the root canal.

Generally one cannot measure the voltage coming from a root canal tooth. However, one can measure the voltage coming from a tooth if it has metal in the form of a filling or crown. Teeth, like the rest of cells, are designed to run at -20 to -25 millivolts. You can take a voltmeter that measures in

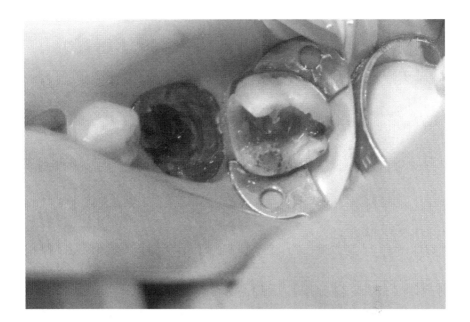

millivolts. Place one electrode on the cheek and one on the metal of the tooth. If you measure more than 100 millivolts, either that tooth or one of its neighbors is infected.

I have a friend that is an oncologist. I looked at 20 of his cancer patients. What I found was that 70% of these patients had a root canal in the same acupuncture meridian as their primary cancer. All but one of the rest had an infected crown in the same meridian as their primary cancer.

In my own practice, I have seen only two patients where I could not find a dental connection to the meridian associated with their cancer. One was a heavy smoker.

These numbers are too small to prove the connection between dental infections and cancer. We can only hope that someone will fund a large study to prove or disprove the connection. In the meantime, it makes sense to remove infections from your teeth and jaws.

We find a similar connection between chronic diseases and dental infections just as Weston Price, DDS described in

Measure Voltage from Dental Fillings that are Metal

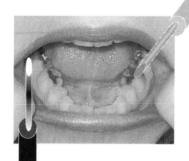
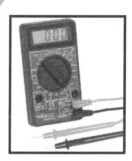

Put black probe on cheek and red on filling. Any measurement above 20 millivolts is abnormal.

1939. The majority of patients I see that have been sick for years have dental infections and most improve dramatically when the infection is removed from their teeth and surrounding bones by appropriate dental intervention. Unfortunately, dentists are routinely harassed by their dental boards if they remove amalgam fillings and root canal teeth based on this science. Therefore it is difficult to find dentists to help you when you are sick from your teeth.

In my experience, most diseases that are called "auto-immune" are caused from a hidden infection. Most of the time it is a dental infection. So-called "auto-immune" diseases often resolve after removing a root canal tooth (or teeth) and infections from under crowns and fillings.

"The idea that inflammatory diseases are caused by an infection is not new. Shortly after World II, Dr. Thomas McPherson Brown of the Rockefeller Institute, isolated tiny bacteria called mycoplasma from the joints of a rheumatoid arthritis (RA) patient.

Claiming to observe the mycoplasma triggering an immune response in animals and humans, Brown developed an antibody test and then announced he'd found the primary cause of RA. Brown also reported positive responses from patients treated with minocycline, an antibiotic used against mycoplasma.

Over the years, thousands of patients were reportedly helped by Brown's treatment. In addition, numerous scientific papers showed a guilt-by-association link between bacteria and inflammation. But Brown continually faced opposition from doctors who argued that inflammatory diseases are the result of an autoimmune problem (i.e., a faulty immune system attacking its own tissues)." http://www.thescavenger.net/ health/inflammatory-diseases-may-be-caused-by-bacteria-74897.html

5 The Bowling Ball Syndrome

In traditional Western medicine it is taught that the cranial bones fuse in childhood. However, it has been taught by Osteopathic doctors since 1874 that the cranial bones move in a rhythmic pattern.

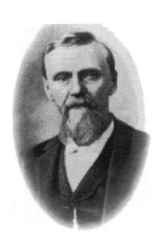

Andrew Taylor Still, MD was a frontier doctor. He wasn't satisfied with the medicine he practiced, particularly when his own children died. He developed the concept of the importance of the movement of the spine. He established Osteopathic Medicine in 1874. The American School of Osteopathy in Kirksville, MO awarded the first 18 diplomas in March, 1894.

According to a school statement, "Osteopathy is the knowledge of the structure, relation and function of each part of the human body applied to the adjustment or correction of whatever interferes with the harmonious operation of the same." George V. Webster, D.O. 1921.

William G. Sutherland, DO developed Cranial Osteopathy. He developed the concept of the respiratory mechanism of the nervous system:

Five Phenomena of the Primary Respiratory Mechanism

1. The central nervous system (brain and spinal cord) has an inherent rhythmic motion.
2. The cerebrospinal fluid (CSF) fluctuates, or moves back and forth in a relatively closed container, the central nervous system.
3. The membranes in the head, called dura mater, surround the bones, comprise major veins in the head, and are essentially continuous with the brain. The dural membranes appear like 3 attached sickles, forming a "tripod" of support for the brain and the skull. They limit and control the slight motion in the bones of the head, and the whole mechanism involving the cranium through the sacrum. The membranes surround the spinal cord like a large cylinder and are anchored firmly to the base of the skull and the sacrum thus forming a core link between the 2 structures.
4. There are 26 bones in the head and they are all in slight rhythmic motion along with the CNS, CSF, membranes, and sacrum. These bones all fit together like the gears of a watch and influence each other.
5. Since the dura mater is attached to the base of the skull and the sacrum (tailbone), as previously

mentioned, the motion of the cranial mechanism is transmitted to the sacrum. The cranium and the sacrum work together as a unit.

Some credit Rollin Becker, DO with the development of the concept of a craniosacral pump. Rollin E. Becker (1910-1996) grew up in an osteopathic household. His father, Arthur D. Becker, D.O. was a prominent and respected osteopath, who served on the faculty with Dr. Andrew Taylor Still and later was dean of two osteopathic colleges. Rollin graduated from the American School of Osteopathy (later renamed the Kirksville College of Osteopathic Medicine) in 1934, and following a few years in Oklahoma, he moved to Michigan, where he practiced for thirteen years.

Rollin Becker, DO

http://www.stillnesspress.com /doc/rollin_becker.htm

In 1944, after about a decade in Michigan, he met William Garner Sutherland, D.O. and in 1948, he first served on the teaching faculty at one of Dr. Sutherland's courses.

Dr. Becker moved to Texas in 1949, where he practiced until 1989. Throughout that time, he continued to serve Dr. Sutherland and his work. Dr. Becker was the president, from 1962 through 1979, of the Sutherland Cranial Teaching Foundation, an educational organization dedicated to perpetuating the teachings of W. G. Sutherland.

In the years following Dr. Sutherland's death in 1954, Dr. Becker played a crucial role in keeping his work alive. He went on to inspire generations of osteopathic teachers and students. http://stillnesspress.com/doc/rollin_becker.htm

John Upledger, DO, a student of Sutherland and a contemporary of Becker, helped develop the science of Craniosacral Therapy in 1975. He also began studies that prove that the cranial bones move with the pulse of the nervous system.

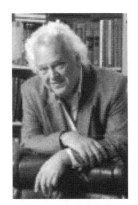

Radiographic Evidence of Cranial Bone Mobility Sheryl Lynn Oleski, B.S.; Gerald H. Smith, D.D.S.; William T. Crow, D.O. From: Cranio: The Journal of Craniomandibular Practice; January 2002, V20N1, pp. 34.

Cranial Bone Movement

HEISEY R; ADAMS T; JOURNAL OF THE AMERICAN OSTEOPATHIC ASSOCIATION; Adams T, Heisey RS, Smith MC, Briner BJ Parietal bone mobility in the anesthetized cat [see comments] In: J Am Osteopath Assoc (1992 May) 92(5): 599-600, 603-10, 615-22 ISSN: 0003-0287

To quantify parietal bone motion in reference to the medial sagittal suture, a newly developed instrument was attached to the surgically exposed skull of anesthetized

adult cats. The instrument differentiated between lateral and rotational parietal bone movements around the fulcrum of the suture. Bone movement was produced by external forces applied to the skull and by changes in intracranial pressure associated with induced hypercapnia, intravenous injections of norepinephrine, and controlled injections of artificial cerebrospinal fluid into the lateral cerebral ventricle. Responses varied considerably among test animals.

Generally, lateral head compression caused sagittal suture closure, small inward rotation of the parietal bones, increased intraventricular pressure, transient apnea, and unstable systemic arterial blood pressure. Graded increases in intracranial volume produced stepped increases in pressure, lateral expansion at the sagittal suture, and outward rotation of the parietal bones. We attribute variations in animal response largely to differences in intracranial and suture compliance among them. Cranial suture compliance may be an important factor in defining total cranial compliance.

Craniosacral Pump

The dura attaches over the sphenoid, down the spine and to the sacrum. This forms a closed hydraulic system. There is a switch in the central joint (medial sagittal suture) that controls formation of cerebrospinal fluid. When the skull bones touch, the switch is on and fluid is deposited inside the dura. This causes the dural balloon to expand.

The Dura over the Sphenoid, Down the Spine and to the Sacrum Forms the CranioSacral Pump

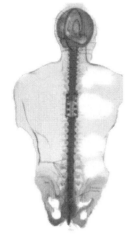
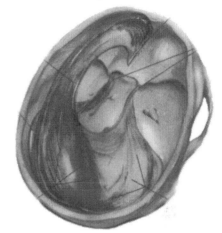

Eventually, this pulls the skull bones apart and the switch is opened. This discontinues the formation of cerebrospinal fluid.

Soon the cerebrospinal fluid leaks out of the dural balloon via the veins and the dural balloon becomes smaller. This allows the skull bones to come back into contact. This reactivates the switch causing fluid to again be produced. This re-expands the dural balloon until again the bones separate causing the switch to open and fluid production to cease.

As this process continues, there forms a vortex movement of fluid inside the dural balloon moving cerebrospinal fluid and its nourishment around the brain and down the spinal cord.

Whenever fluid moves within a magnetic field, electrons are generated. For example, when a river runs downhill within the earth's magnetic field called the Schumann field, electrons are added to the water. This is accompanied by the formation of a vortex in the middle of the river. Each of us has experienced walking in a stream and feeling the vortex of water moving against our ankles as we approach the center of the stream. This same phenomenon is happening within our dural balloon.

The upper part of the dural balloon is attached to the sphenoid bone of the skull. The lower part of the dural balloon is attached to the sacrum. When it pulses, it forms the Craniosacral Pump. As the sphenoid and sacrum move, the cerebrospinal fluid circulates through the brain and spinal cord.

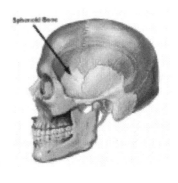

When the sphenoid is de-centered and jammed, the pump stops. The nervous system must function with stagnant cerebrospinal fluid.

The "Bowling Ball" syndrome was described by Robert Boyd, DO from Ireland. (An Introduction to Bio Cranial Therapy; Bio Cranial Institute; Charlotte, NC). Boyd stated that the head weighs about the same as a bowling ball. Because it weighs so much, the body will always put the upper cervical vertebra under the center of gravity of the head to keep the head upright. When the sphenoid bone (keystone) is

Robert Boyd, DO and Wife, Vera

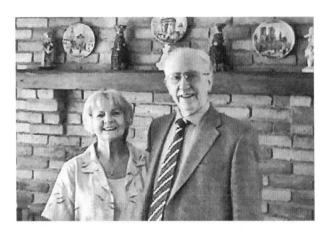

61

moved, the other cranial bones follow. This moves the center of gravity of the skull causing the compensatory changes:

6. The two sides of the face are asymmetrical.
7. The jaw moves to one side causing TMJ
8. One eyelid is droopy (ptosis) and the opposite cheek is flattened.
9. One ear canal is lower than the other.
10. Obstruction of the ocular canal can increase intraocular pressure and decrease visual fields.
11. Kinking of the Eustachian tubes can lead to increased ear infections.
12. Sinus obstruction.
13. Nasal obstruction.
14. Snoring.
15. C1-2 move to one side causing persistent headaches and neckaches.

16. The entire spine is curved causing extrusion of disks.
17. One shoulder is higher than the other making one arm seem short.
18. One scapula is higher than the other giving pain in the interscapular area during driving and other use of the arms.
19. The pelvis is rotated giving low back pain and disk extrusion.
20. The rotated pelvis makes one leg relatively shorter than the other. This places more weight on one hip-knee-ankle making those joints wear out.
21. The shift of weight to one side makes one clumsier.
22. The locking of the craniosacral pump causes the entire nervous system to use stagnant cerebrospinal fluid resulting in a general decrease in its function.
23. Migraine headaches.

Trapezius Muscle

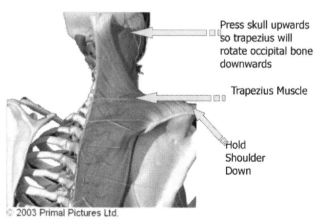

Press skull upwards so trapezius will rotate occipital bone downwards

Trapezius Muscle

Hold Shoulder Down

© 2003 Primal Pictures Ltd.

Boyd described the Bowling Ball Syndrome in osteopathic terms. He developed a mechanical means of attempting to correct the Bowling Ball Syndrome that he called Bio Cranial Therapy. It involves placing one hand under the occiput and pinning the shoulder to the table. The head is moved in a certain arc to the maximum extension of the trapezius muscle and then a little farther. This pulls backward on the occipital bone. The occipital bone is attached to the sphenoid. This re-centers the sphenoid.

NeuroCranial Restructuring

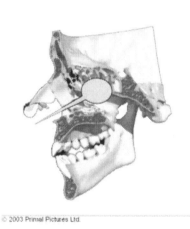

© 2003 Primal Pictures Ltd.

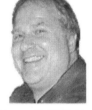

Dean Howell, ND teaches the placement of a balloon through the nostril and under the sphenoid to move it.

Dean Howell of Seattle teaches placing a balloon through a nostril into the pharynx under the sphenoid. When the balloon is inflated quickly, it moves the sphenoid upward and re-centers it. He calls this Neuro-Cranial Restructuring.

I was amazed by the results of correcting the Bowling Ball Syndrome when it was demonstrated to me by Doug Hays,

DC! As I began to consider how it worked, I found a different perspective than the one taught by Dr. Boyd.

If one stacks up stones to form an arch, the piece inserted at the top of the arch is known as the keystone. The keystone, because of its shape, keeps the arch standing by causing the blocks in the arch to push against each other. When extra weight is applied to the top of the arch, the keystone

Keystone

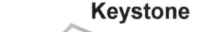

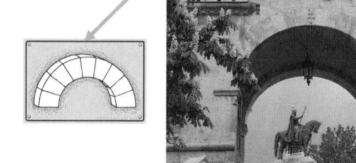

helps to direct the force sideways through the other blocks.

The sphenoid bone is the keystone for the skull. The other cranial bones rest on the sphenoid. The position of the sphenoid (keystone) dictates the position of all other skull bones. The sphenoid bone is often moved by trauma (birth trauma and accidents). Thus the position of the sphenoid bone dictates the center of gravity of the skull. When it shifts causing the other cranial bones to shift as well, it moves the center of gravity of the skull. This causes the brain to tell the neck, particularly the upper cervical vertebra, to move to get under the center of gravity of the skull so it won't fall over. This dictate from the brain changes the anatomical alignment of the whole body!

Bowling Ball Syndrome

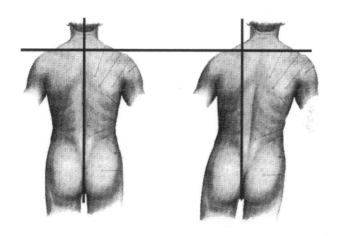

Alexander Revenko, MD is a Russian neurologist involved with the SCENAR device. He described a technique using the SCENAR in acute settings to pulse the

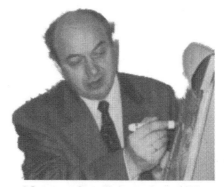

Alexander Revenko, MD

trapezius = called it "Little Wings".

I described a technique using the SCENAR in default settings to create a strong contraction of the trapezius to simulate Bio-Cranial Therapy. It is more complete and less painful than Bio-Cranial Therapy. The technique involves placing the SCENAR in the same location as Little Wings on the side of the neck. One then increases the power until one gets an intense spasm of the trapezius for five seconds. This pulls intently on the occipital bone. Through its attachment to the sphenoid, the sphenoid is re-centered. This is performed on both sides of the neck to be certain the

Autonomic "Reset Button"

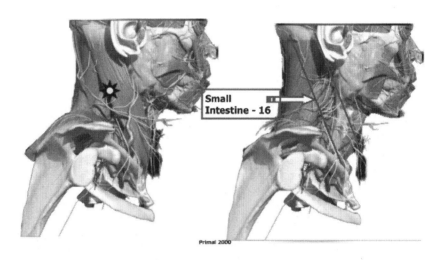

Small Intestine - 16

Primal 2000

sphenoid is centered.

The mechanical correction of the Bowling Ball with the SCENAR is very annoying to the patient. I found that the same correction could be achieved energetically with the Tennant Biomodulator®. This is done at a power setting that is not annoying to the patient using the mode called Infinity. It is the preferred method.

Immediately after correcting the Bowling Ball with the Tennant Biomodulator, the ears become level and the pelvic rotation is gone. It takes about ½ to one hour for the cranial bones to completely re-center and the ptosis to disappear. It takes 24 hours for the shoulders to become even. The craniosacral pump begins pumping immediately, but it often is irregular for about one hour. This can be tested by having the patient stand with their eyes closed. Before correcting the Bowling Ball, they will stand very still. After correction, they begin to sway back and forth about twelve times per minute.

In over ninety percent of the patients, the correction is complete and permanent unless another head trauma occurs. In those patients with low total body voltage, it slips back out and must be re-corrected.

Brain Waves and the Bowling Ball

The brain has four "gears" like an automobile:
1. Delta = sleep
2. Theta = not awake, not asleep
3. Alpha = daydreaming
4. Beta = thinking

Whenever the brain is malfunctioning (infection, trauma, metabolic), it produces excess second gear (Theta waves) as an adaptive mechanism to help prevent seizures. This adaptive mechanism is both helpful (prevents seizures) and harmful (makes you function in second gear). (NATIONAL HEAD INJURY SYLLABUS, HEAD INJURY FRONTIERS, Margaret Ayers, PAGE 380, 1987)

Most EEG devices apply Fourier mathematics to the data before it is presented. The Neuropathways EEG device developed by Margaret Ayers shows actual data 1/1000 second after it occurs in the brain. Since you see the real data, you can see patterns of infection, closed head injury, open head injury, glucose metabolism insufficiency, and allergy. In addition, one can see the average voltage for each type of wave. Normal for Theta and Beta is two microvolts. (http://www.neuropathways.com/default.htm)

Nineteen patients were examined with the Neuropathways EEG device before and after correcting the Bowling Ball Syndrome electronically. The reduction of Theta waves ranged from 2-50% with an average reduction of 15% with one treatment.

Autonomic Nervous System

The autonomic nervous system consists of two parts, the sympathetic and parasympathetic systems. The sympathetic system is known as the "fight or flight" system and the parasympathetic system is known as the "eat, sleep, and heal" system.

Assume there is a deer in the forest. He thinks he hears a mountain lion. His sympathetic system turns on and his parasympathetic system turns off. As the sympathetic system activates, his pupils dilate, his ears stand erect, his bronchioles open wider, blood moves from his G.I. tract to his muscles effectively shutting down the digestive system, and his muscles are at attention while he figures out if he is going to be required to fight the lion or runaway. As you can see, during sympathetic -- on, the things necessary to see better, hear better move more air into and out of the lungs, and put all senses of high alert are effected. At the same time, the digestive system is shut down so its resources can be transferred to the muscles.

Now assume the lion did not show up. The sympathetic system turns down and the parasympathetic system turns back on. Pupils go back to normal size, ears lay down, the bronchioles relax, and the digestive system turns back on. The deer munches on some grass, takes a nap, and starts the healing process.

An important thing to notice is that the digestive system cannot work effectively while you are in sympathetic -- on.

A significant difference between the deer and humans is that humans often get stuck in sympathetic -- on. While in this mode, the digestive system doesn't function well, sleep is difficult, and healing cannot occur.

When you have the bowling ball syndrome, you are stuck in sympathetic -- on.

Almost everyone suffering from chronic illness has the bowling ball syndrome. One of the amazing things that happens when you correct it is that it balances the sympathetic and parasympathetic systems. Thus, not only does the correction cause your posture and anatomical alignment to be corrected, it takes you out of sympathetic -- on and balances your autonomic nervous system. This allows you to enter parasympathetic -- on with the ability to have normal digestion, sleep better, and heal.

I know of no other therapy that will do this. The five-minute correction of the bowling ball syndrome benefits patients more than any other therapy I know of. It is important that each patient with chronic disease be checked to see that their bowling ball has been corrected every day. It is easy for people to learn how to correct the bowling ball syndrome for themselves using the Tennant BioModulator.

6 Nitric Oxide

Nitrous oxide, commonly known as laughing gas or sweet air, is a chemical compound with the formula N2O. It is used in surgery and dentistry for its anesthetic and analgesic effects. It is known as "laughing gas" due to the euphoric effects of inhaling it.

Nitric Oxide (NO) is a gas that serves as a signaling molecule in every cell in the body.
1. It causes arteries and bronchioles to expand
2. It allows brain cells to communicate with each other
3. It causes immune cells to kill bacteria and cancer cells

Nitric Oxide was discovered in 1772 by a British man named Joseph Priestly, who referred to it as "nitrous air." When he discovered this, it was a colorless and gas and a toxic gas. Nitric Oxide continued to receive the label of being a toxic gas and an air pollutant until over two hundred years later, in 1987, when it was proven to be naturally produced by the body of mammals, including humans. 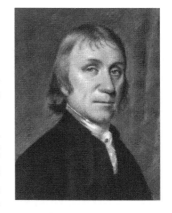 http:// itech.dickinson.edu/chemistry/?p=260

In 1998, the Nobel Prize in Physiology and Medicine was awarded jointly to Robert F. Furchgott, Louis J.

Ignarro and Ferid Murad for their discoveries that nitric oxide is a signaling molecule in the cardiovascular system.

In mammals, NO is an important cellular messenger molecule involved in many physiological and pathological processes. Low levels of NO production are important in protecting an organ such as the liver from ischemic damage. However, sustained levels of increased NO production result in direct tissue damage and contribute to the vascular collapse associated with septic shock, whereas chronic expression of NO is associated with various carcinomas and inflammatory conditions including juvenile diabetes, multiple sclerosis, arthritis and ulcerative colitis.

Altitude Sickness	Heart attack
Arteries-flexible	Hypertension
Artery-plaques	Incontinence
Asthma	Insomnia
Bacterial Infections	Kidney Disease
Blood clots	Macular Degeneration
Cancer	Memory Loss
Cholesterol	Obesity
COPD	Osteoarthritis
Depression	Prematures
Diabetes	Sickle cell
Dementia	Stomach Ulcers
Eclampsia	Stress
Erectile Dysfunction	Stroke
Glaucoma	Sun Damage

As you can see in the table, lack of NO (nitric oxide) is a controlling factor in many illnesses that plague us.

On the average, Americans lose 10% of the ability to make NO for every decade of life. This loss of NO plays a significant role in the development of the diseases noted in the table.

NO is biosynthesized from L-arginine, oxygen and NADPH by various nitric oxide synthase (NOS) enzymes. Reduction of inorganic nitrate may also serve to make nitric oxide. There are several things that interfere with this process causing us to lose our ability to make NO.

The process of making NO requires calcium, copper, iron, magnesium, manganese, molybdenum, nickel, selenium, and zinc. It also requires Vitamin B1 (thiamine), Vitamin B2 (riboflavin), Vitamin B3 (niacin or niacinamide), Vitamin B5 (pantothenic acid), Vitamin B6 (pyridoxine), Vitamin B7 (biotin), Vitamin B9 (folic acid), Vitamin B12 (various cobalamins), Vitamin C, Vitamin K1, and Vitamin K2.

Arginine is synthesized from the amino acid citrulline by the sequential action of the cytosolic enzymes argininosuccinate synthetase (ASS) and argininosuccinate lyase (ASL).

Arginine is a conditionally nonessential amino acid, meaning most of the time it can be manufactured by the human body, and does not need to be obtained directly through the diet. The biosynthetic pathway however does not produce sufficient arginine, and some must still be consumed through diet. Individuals who have poor nutrition or certain physical conditions may be advised to increase their intake of foods containing arginine. Arginine is found in a wide variety of foods. Animal sources: dairy products (e.g. cottage cheese, ricotta, milk, yogurt, whey protein drinks), beef, pork (e.g. bacon, ham), gelatin , poultry (e.g. chicken and turkey light meat), wild game (e.g. pheasant, quail), seafood (e.g. halibut, lobster, salmon, shrimp, snails, tuna). Plant sources: wheat germ and flour, buckwheat, granola, oatmeal, peanuts, nuts (coconut, pecans, cashews, walnuts, almonds, Brazil nuts, hazelnuts, pine nuts), seeds (pumpkin, sesame, sunflower), chick peas, cooked soybeans, Phalaris canariensis (canary seed or ALPISTE). wikipedia

A more recent finding is that NO is also made from nitrates and nitrites. Nitrates turn into nitrites in the body which then turn into NO. Don't be confused by the generally held opinion that nitrates and nitrites are poisonous. In the 1950's to the 1970's, there was found an association between nitrates, nitrites and cancer. However, these were Relative Risks as we have discussed in the chapter on medical studies. You will recall that high Relative Risks can really be meaningless and that one should just examine Absolute Risks.

In a summary report, the World Cancer Research Fund and the American Institute for Cancer Research recommended avoiding processed meats based on a meta-analysis showing a link between processed meats and colorectal cancer with a Relative Risk of 21%. In 1994, the National Cancer Institute stated that Relative Risks below 200 percent were not strong enough to make public policy pronouncements about risk factors!

People that eat vegetable diets to lower blood pressure consume nitrates and nitrites five times the amount higher than that proposed by the World Health Organization!. The amount of nitrates and nitrites in your saliva after you eat a spinach salad is much higher than that recommended by the scientific "experts". Does spinach and your saliva cause cancer? Not

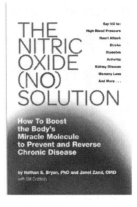

likely. Moreover, the amount of nitrates and nitrites in breast milk is higher than in any other food or beverage!

For this reason, a NO Index has been created. It takes into account:
1. The total amount of NO creating nitrate and nitrite in a food
2. The ORAC (oxygen radical absorption capacity) of a food---its amount of antioxidants (electron donors) available to protect the NO

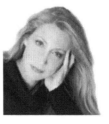

NO Index: This table is from The Nitric Oxide Solution by Nathan S. Bryan, PhD and Janet Zand, OMD. You really must get this book.

        One of the things that is new about NO is our ability to easily measure it. Although there are over 1000 medical research studies available about NO, few doctors even think about it because we haven't had a way to measure it. Most doctors therefore have no idea how to correct it.

Arginine food sources	Arginine content
Plant products	(grams /100 gram of food)
Peanuts, Spanish	3.13
Peanuts	3.09
Almond nuts	2.47
Seeds, sunflower seed kernels, dried	2.40
Walnuts, English	2.28
Hazelnuts	2.21
Lentils, raw	2.17
Brazilnuts	2.15
Cashew nuts	2.12
Pistachio nuts	2.03
Flax seed	1.93
Beans, kidney, all types, mature seeds, raw	1.46
Pecan nuts	1.18
Beans, French, mature seeds, raw	1.17
Soybeans, green, raw	1.04
Tofu, extra firm, prepared with nigari	0.66
Wheat flour, whole-grain	0.64
Garlic, raw	0.63
Muffins, blueberry, toaster-type	0.30
Onion, raw	0.10
Chocolate syrup	0.09
Animal products	
Fish, tuna, light, canned in oil, drained solids	1.74
Chicken, broilers or fryers, giblets, raw	1.19
Salmon, Atlantic, farmed, raw	1.19
Shrimp, mixed species, raw	1.18
Egg, yolk, raw, fresh	1.10
Egg, whole, raw	0.82
Egg, white, raw, fresh	0.65
Pork, fresh, separable fat, raw	0.56
Milk, whole, 3.25% milkfat	0.08

A test strip is now available that only requires one to spit on the strip. In one minute, it tells you your levels!   See https://secure.neogenis.com/product-listing.html

There are a lot of supplement companies selling products to increase your NO. However, most of them contain l-arginine. This can be a problem because most people that need to correct their NO levels are over the age of 40, have hypertension, obesity, diabetes, high cholesterol, and/or are smokers. **Such people should not take l-arginine as it can actually increase their risk of a heart attack!**

A study at Johns Hopkins was started giving l-arginine to people that had suffered a heart attack. They found that it didn't improve cardiac ejection fractions or arterial stiffness,   However, six people in the l-arginine group died of another heart attack while none died in the placebo group. Therefore the study was stopped and it was recommended that l-arginine NOT be given to anyone that has had a heart attack.

Nitric oxide is synthesized by nitric oxide synthase (NOS). There are three isoforms of the NOS enzyme:
1. Endothelial (eNOS):   Signaling molecule-- Calcium dependent; produces low levels of gas as a cell signaling molecule
2. Neuronal (nNOS):   Signaling molecule-- Calcium dependent; produces low levels of gas as a cell signaling molecule
3. Inducible (Immune System) (iNOS)--Calcium Independent; produces large amounts of gas which can be cytotoxic

Nitric oxide secreted as an immune response is secreted as free radicals and is toxic to bacteria; the mechanism for this includes DNA damage. In response, however, many bacterial pathogens have evolved mechanisms for nitric oxide resistance.

If a person doesn't have the cofactors to make NO from l-arginine, it can increase the amount of cytotoxic compounds made by the immune system pathway. This is similar to converting the thyroid hormone T-4 to T-3. If you don't have the vitamins and minerals necessary for the conversion, you make the fake hormone RT3 that keeps your cells from working correctly. If you don't have the cofactors necessary to convert l-arginine, it can be harmful to you! Taking citrulline instead of l-arginine helps solve this.

Another problem is the presence of fluoride. When fluoride is present, it converts NO into the toxic and destructive nitric acid. NO will react with fluorine, chlorine, and bromine to form the XNO species, known as the nitrosyl halides, such as nitrosyl chloride. Nitrosyl iodide can form but is an extremely short-lived species and tends to reform I2.

$$2\ NO + Cl2 \longrightarrow 2\ NOCl.$$

Nitrosyl fluoride reacts with water to form nitrous acid, which then forms nitric acid:

$$NOF + H2O \longrightarrow HNO2 + HF$$
$$3\ HNO2 \longrightarrow HNO3 + 2\ NO + H2O$$

Being a powerful oxidizing agent (electron stealer), nitric acid reacts violently with many organic materials and the reactions may be explosive. wikipedia

An often overlooked fact is that the amino acids in the foods listed are only available if you have stomach acid to convert the proteins that are in the listed foods into amino acids. If you don't have stomach acid, the amino acids are not available and you can't make NO. Remember that to make stomach acid, you need Vitamin B1, iodine, and zinc. Without stomach acid, you can't absorb zinc even if you take it, so you have to take a Betaine tablet with the zinc so it will be absorbed.

So---remember to correct your stomach acid and eat your green vegetables. Correct your vitamin and mineral levels so you can make nitric oxide. It can help prevent glaucoma, macular degeneration, heart attacks, strokes, diabetes, and all the other maladies listed and even improve or restore your sex life!

7 Humic/Fulvic Acid

Fungus and the Planet

Most of us think of fungus as something disgusting in the same category as insects. It's everywhere but you try to avoid it (with the exception of the mushrooms you put on your salad and steak). The reality is that fungus plays a

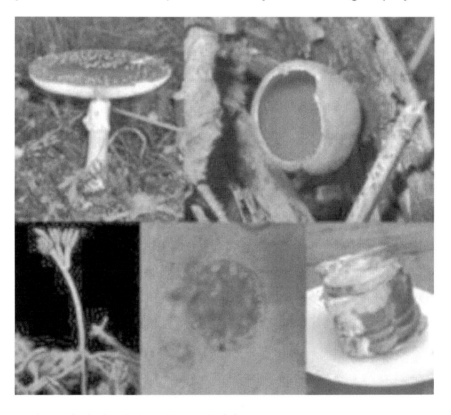

major role in both health and sickness.

Fungus is the kingdom of organisms that includes yeasts, rusts, molds, and mushrooms. Fungus has characteristics of both plants and animals. They contain cell membranes surrounding a nucleus (like an animal cell) whereas bacteria have no nucleus. They contain no chlorophyll to make energy like plants but they create toxins and enzymes to consume organic material from plants or animals. Fungus reproduces by spores (one-celled reproductive units) that are asexual. Spores cannot be damaged even with extreme heat and can lay dormant for years. They produce energy without the use of oxygen (fermentation) (anaerobic).

The Role of Fungus on the Planet

The reason fungus is present on the earth is to decompose dead organic material. If it were not for fungus, we would all be over our heads in dead leaves and dead animals!

Think about a leaf growing on a tree. It is covered with fungal spores that are doing nothing. They are suppressed by the voltage of the leaf. Since the leaf is living, it contains voltage. If the tree becomes sick, the voltage of the leaf can drop. However, when the season comes for the leaf to drop to the ground, the voltage in the leaf drops significantly. As it does so, this signals the fungus to "wake up" and convert from a spore to its adult form. This fungus does what fungus is designed to do. It converts the leaf to its component parts of vitamins, minerals, and amino acids. These become what we call "dirt" or "soil". The scientific name given this dirt is "humic acid". Humic acid is not a single acid like hydrochloric acid. Rather it is the combination of the components of what used to be a leaf.

A small portion of the humic acid is called "fulvic acid". Fulvic is the key that opens cell membranes so that nutrition can pass into cells.

Now a seed is blown into the dirt. The seed needs nutrients. The fulvic acid in the soil opens the membranes of the seed and allow humic to flow into the seed. If the necessary water is present, it begins to grow. It grows into a plant containing vitamins, minerals, amino acids along with humic and fulvic acid.

The human pulls the plant and eats it. Now the human contains the humic, fulvic, vitamins, minerals, and amino acids needed for cells to work. The fulvic opens the cells of the human so nutrition can flow into the cell. The human is now able to make new cells and grow and repair itself until death finally occurs and the human is returned to dirt the same way the dead leaf was. Fungus renders the human into dirt with its component parts.

The problem of illness starts with pesticides. The pesticides that farmers put on the soil kills the fungus. That means that there is no longer a process to continuously provide soil with humic and fulvic. Eventually the plants won't grow. Then the farmer adds fertilizer so the plants will grow. The fertilizer contains potassium, phosphorous, and nitrogen. These make the plant grow, but they are deficient in vitamins, minerals, amino acids, humic and fulvic. We pull this plant and eat it, but such plants have almost no nutrition. And since these plants don't have humic and fulvic, eventually the human becomes deficient in them as well. Without fulvic, the nutrients taken can't enter the cells and so the cell struggles for nutrition. Disease isn't far behind.

Fungus and Disease

Just as leaves and dead animals are destroyed by fungus as the voltage falls, so the human is filled with fungus. As long as the human's voltage is normal, the fungus is dormant. However, if hypothyroidism, dental infections, lack of stomach acid, and toxins such as fluoride, chlorine, aspartame, Splenda, MSG, antibiotics, and many others that are in our food supply and environment drop our voltage, the fungus wakes up and begins to do what fungus is designed to do. It destroys our cells.

There are about 70,000 species of fungi, 200 of which cause disease in humans. The number of human fungal infections is directly related to the amount of antibiotics (fungal derivatives) consumed by the patient. The more antibiotics consumed means more secondary fungal infections. Antibiotics are consumed as medical therapy and in our food as most meat-producing animals and birds are given antibiotics to increase and speed-up their growth.

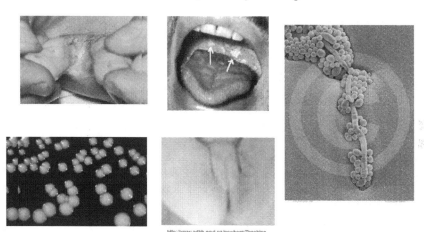

http://www.adhb.govt.nz/newborn/Teaching

The yeast Candida albicans has become the fourth most frequent hospital infection. Eight variations of Candida cause disease in man. Candida usually enter the body via the intestine when the guts' good bacteria are killed by antibiotics.

In the 1930's Royal Rife identified material that could be filtered from bacteria through a ceramic filters that only allowed passage of things smaller than 300 microns. He called them "filterable bacteria" because they could cause disease in animals. Particles smaller than 300 microns are now considered to be fungal spores or viruses. Bacteria are around 1000 microns (1,000,000 nanometers) in diameter.

Fungi and bacteria compete with each other for their food supply. Good bacteria in the gut help retard the growth of fungi. Fungi produce "antibiotics" in an effort to kill the bacteria. Pharmaceutical companies use fungi to make antibiotics like penicillin.

Examples of Diseases Caused or Aggravated by Fungi
1. Cancer
2. Migraines
3. Crohn's Disease
4. GERD
5. Asthma
6. Chronic Fatigue
7. Leukemia
8. Lymphoma
9. High Cholesterol
10. Hypertension
11. Diabetes
12. Infertility
13. ADHD

Koch's Postulates Remove Fungus from Consideration in Most Infectious Disease

In 1862, Robert Koch, MD, a German doctor discovered the tuberculosis bacteria, Mycobacterium tuberculosis. Notice that its name means "fungal bacteria". Koch developed the standard to determine the cause of infectious diseases. Koch's Postulates say that a microbe must be:
Found in an animal with a disease.
Isolated and grown in culture.
Injected into a healthy animal to produce the disease.
Recovered from the injected animal and found to be the same as the first one.

Fungi are mostly unable to fulfill Koch's Postulates because:

1. They exist in many different forms (spores, mycelia, with and without cells walls, etc.)
2. They are very difficult to culture. They can hide for years as spores until conditions are favorable for them to grow.
3. There are no rapid diagnostic tests to confirm the presence of fungus in the body except live blood analysis with phase contrast or dark field microscopes---not generally used in traditional medicine..
4. Filterable microbes include not only viruses but fungal spores (they may be the same thing)!

Fungus and Cancer

1840's: Louis Pasteur claims each disease is caused by a single external organism.
1840's: Antoine Beauchamp found that microorganisms change from one form to another (pleomorphism).
1840's: Claude Bernard felt that the body's internal environment controlled disease (voltage?).
1872-1968: Gunther Enderlein felt fungi changed from normal to pathogenic inside the body according to the environment.
1899: Dr. Bra (French) announced, "The parasite is fungus-like and is certainly the specific agent of cancer." Nothing more was heard of his announcement.
1925: Dr John Nuzum of Chicago reported consistently culturing organisms that changed shapes from breast cancer.
1925: Dr. Michael Scott of Montana found organism in cancer that changed from stage to stage as coccus, rod, and "spore sac".
1931: Otto Warburg receives Nobel Prize for showing that cancer cells get energy by fermentation the same way fungi do.
1947: Virginia Livingston-Wheeler cultures microbes from all cancers studied.

1950: Drs. Livingston-Wheeler, Wuerthele-Caspe, Jackson, and Diller remove microbes from cancer tissue and use them to cause cancer in animals. They then re-cultured the microbes from the tumors of the animals.
1960: Aflatoxin, (naturally occurring mycotoxins that are produced by many species of Aspergillus, a fungus, most notably Aspergillus flavus) , is discovered in England. It caused the death of thousands of turkeys and was found to cause liver cancer in humans.
1976: Kurt Olbrich develops microscope that can see things <100 nm. He can find fungus in the blood of all patients with cancer two years before they can be diagnosed with CAT scans, MRI scans, etc.
1997: Dr. Mark Bielski states lymphocytic leukemia is always associated with Candida albicans.
1999: Meinolf Karthaus cures leukemia with anti-fungal drugs.
2008: Tullio Simoncini cures cancer with sodium bicarbonate (baking soda) if he can bathe the tumor in it.

An understanding of infectious disease began in the mid 1800's with French scientists Louis Pasteur, Antoine Beauchamp, and Claude Bernard.

★Pasteur believed that each disease was caused by an externally acquired single infectious organism.
★Beauchamp believed that each disease was caused by infectious organisms that are always in our bodies and changing forms from helpful to pathogenic. He was the first to identify small particles that turned into other forms that he called microzymas.
★Bernard believed that the body's internal environment dictated whether infectious disease could occur. He drank a pitcher full of plague bacteria before the medical society to prove it would not harm him.

Prostate Specific Antigen (PSA)

Prostate Specific Antigen is NOT prostate specific! PSA (33-kDa serine protease) is elevated in prostate, breast, ovarian, pancreatic, and colon cancer. PSA is produced by Aspergillus flavus, A. fungigatus, A. oryzae, Ophiostoma piceae, Scedosporium apiospermum (all of the Ascomycete group of fungi). **A high PSA is an indicator of fungus in the blood!**

Kolattukudy found that PSA is a "significant virulence factor in invasive aspergillosis, which increased metastatic spread and mortality".

Aspergillus molds are the major producers of aflatoxin. Aflatoxins are the most potent liver carcinogens in the world.

Catchfly Plant and Cancer

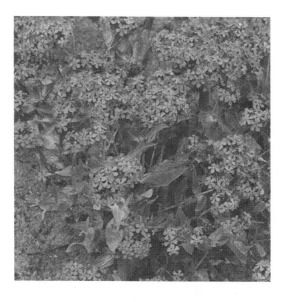

Catchfly plants are any of several plants of the genera Silene and Lychnis, native chiefly to the Northern Hemisphere and having white, pink, red, or purplish flowers and sticky stems and calyxes on which small insects may become stuck. When infected with fungus, the plant's DNA is mixed with fungal DNA so that the fungus takes control of the plant. Instead of producing pollen, the plant begins to produce fungal spores!

The fungus performs a sex-change operation on female catchfly plants, causing them to abort their ovaries and develop stamens -- male sex organs that normally produce pollen. And whatever the gender of its host, U. violacea secretly transforms stamens into spore factories. Dusted with spores instead of pollen, insects lured to the early, long-lasting blossoms unwittingly spread the fungal infection to the next cluster of catchfly they visit.

It apparently has not been studied. However, if this same thing happens in humans, it would explain what is normally called "random mutation" of DNA in cancer patients. Thus as voltage drops, fungus in the human wakes up and infects human cells. It could be that the fungus then takes over the DNA changing the cell into a cancer cell. Making more fungus makes more cancer cells. Since the role of fungus is to decompose dead organic material, it performs this role. However, it is accomplished inside an organism that is still alive until it finally kills the organism.

Fungi in Industry

1. Fungi are used to manufacture:
2. Citric acid (from Aspergillus niger) used in soft drinks
3. Inks
4. Dyeing processes
5. Silvering of mirrors
6. Pharmaceuticals
7. Antibiotics
8. Ephedrine
9. Vitamins
10. Enzymes
11. Alcoholic beverages
12. Bread
13. Cheese

Animal vs. Plant

Animal cells have nuclei and need oxygen for energy production by respiration. Plant cells use carbon dioxide and chlorophyll to make energy and release oxygen. Fungal cells have nuclei but in the yeast form, make energy without oxygen (just like plants) and without chlorophyll (unlike plants) in a process called fermentation.

When you take antibiotics (fungal toxins), they kill bacteria but nothing kills them. The amount of fungal infections in your body is directly related to the amount of antibiotics you have taken.

Candida albicans has become the fourth leading cause of hospital-acquired blood-stream infections. Eight different Candida species infect humans. Probiotics (good bacteria in the gut) compete with fungus for the same food. Probiotics are THE MOST IMPORTANT defense you have against fungal invasion! Fermentation (feeding the fungus) requires sugar and low voltage. **If you crave carbohydrates, you are likely infected with fungus.**

When animals were fed moldy feed, it was noticed that they put on weight faster and in greater amounts! Thus farmers began to give their animals antibiotics (mold products). When you eat farm animals/fish that have been fed fungus, you eat fungus/fungal toxins.

Like other animals, humans put on weight faster when they consume antibiotics either as a prescription medication or in meat from animals that were fed antibiotics.

Patients who are allergic to penicillin have very few antibodies against penicillin in their blood. **People who are allergic to penicillin are filled with fungus/fungal toxins**. A small addition of more fungus (penicillin tablet) causes the body to be overwhelmed with rashes and can lead to death.

Conidia (Spores That Have Lost Cell Membrane and Entered Cells)

1. Conidia (fungal spores without shell) and viruses are very similar:
2. Can only live inside a cell or sac.
3. Trigger disease.
4. Can remain quiescent for years.
5. Can form buds, break off, and infect other cells.

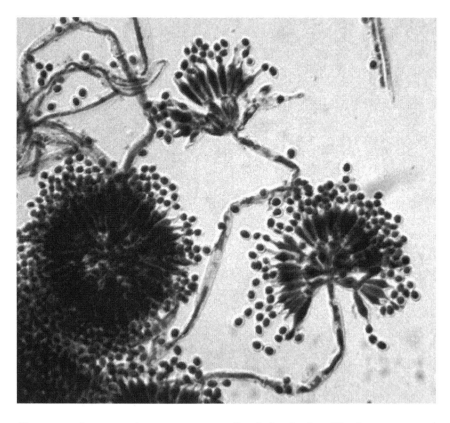

Corn and peanuts are generally infected with fungus and contain the fungal toxin aflatoxin. Penicillin and most antibiotics are fungi that kill or inhibit bacteria. When you take them they kill the bacteria but remain behind in your system.

Taking Antibiotics Increases the Risk of Cancer and Other Diseases

Prior Medication Use And Health History As Risk Factors For Non- Hodgkin's Lymphoma: Preliminary Results From A Case-Control Study In Los Angeles County. Bernstein L, Ross RK; Cancer Res (1992 Oct 1) 52(19 Suppl): 5510s-5515s

Abstract: To determine whether non-Hodgkin's lymphoma (NHL) is related to prior medication use or health history, a population-based case-control study was conducted. A total of 619 male and female residents of Los Angeles County who were diagnosed with NHL between January 1, 1979, and June 30, 1982, were compared to individually age-, race-, and sex- matched neighborhood controls with regard to history of use of 49 different medications, 47 chronic and infectious diseases or other conditions, 15 types of immunizations, and 15 specific allergic reactions.
Based on preliminary analyses, long-term regular use of aspirin and other pain relievers and greater than or equal to 2 months Women who had been immunized against polio by injectable vaccine were at significantly lower risk of NHL than women who had not received this immunization.
Among men, cholera immunization and allergy to nuts and berries were significantly protective. Subjects who had received a yellow fever immunization also had lower NHL risk.

Further analyses of these data will attempt to establish the relative importance of these potential risk factors and to determine whether any are markers of early symptoms of NHL. of treatment with penicillin and other antibiotics were associated with significantly increased risk of Non-Hodgkin's Leukemia.

170

Other drugs associated with greater risk of NHL were use of digitalis and estrogen replacement therapy by women, use of corticosteroids, and greater than or equal to 2 months of use of tranquilizers.

NHL was strongly associated with a prior history of cancer. Cases more frequently reported histories of kidney infections and anemia than did controls; a history of eczema appeared to be protective against NHL.

This study shows the role of pharmaceuticals in lowering voltage, allowing fungus to produce cancer. Once you understand the role of fungus in disease and the role of voltage in controlling fungus, you begin to understand the paradigm that Healing is Voltage.

We see that fungus has the amazing duality of both preventing disease by creating humic and fulvic acid to provide nutrition to the cells of living things and to cause disease when it finds that cells have low voltage. When the voltage is low enough, fungus causes cancer. All of this is controlled by voltage because voltage controls oxygen levels and oxygen levels control fungus.

Farming practices of using pesticides and fertilizers create foods that have little nutrition. In addition, they don't contain adequate amounts of humic and fulvic to keep the human that eats these foods healthy.

Humic and Fulvic Supplements

One of the keys to regaining health is to put humic and fulvic acids into the body even when they are missing from our food supply. Otherwise, the nutrition in the food you eat and even the supplements you take have trouble getting into the cells.

I have developed a product called Raw Materials that contains the things necessary to make new cells.

8 Healing Eye Diseases

I have been an ophthalmologist/eye surgeon since 1968. During this time, I have been able to make some contributions to improving the treatment of eye diseases and the results of surgery, particularly cataract surgery. Among my contributions have been:

Outpatient Surgicenters for Eye Surgery
I helped to develop the techniques to move eye surgery from the hospital to the outpatient surgery centers. Among those involved in this effort were Norvell Christy, MD, Douglas Williamson, MD, David McIntyre, MD, Miles Galin, MD, and the gifted anesthesiologist, Monte Hellman, MD that developed the techniques for safe and effective anesthesia for outpatient eye surgery. In 1978, I had been working at Methodist Hospital of Dallas. Many of my eye surgery patients became ill while in the hospital for eye surgery. They couldn't get the same diet they were used to at home. They got their medications at different times. They had trouble sleeping because of the strange beds and constant noises characteristic of hospitals. I began sending my patients home immediately after eye surgery and solved these problems. I could do this because I had developed a water-tight incision. At a meeting of ophthalmologists in the Century Plaza Hotel in Los Angeles, Dave McIntyre, Doug Williamson and I sat eating lunch. We discussed the need for training ophthalmologists how to do outpatient eye surgery. We decided to start the Outpatient Ophthalmic Surgery Society. We wrote the bylaws on napkins and thus

started the efforts to train US surgeons how to perform outpatient eye surgery.

Self-sealing Incisions

In the 1970's, it was common to make a small incision into the eye and then place scissors into the eye to enlarge the incision to remove the cataract. Large sutures of silk were used to close the wound. These incisions easily leaked fluid if there was pressure on the eye or if the patient sneezed or strained when they became constipated.

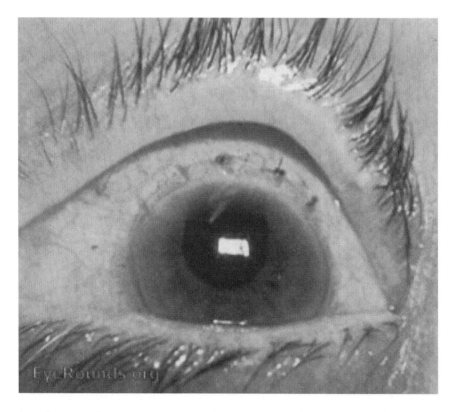

In the early 1970's, I had begun making a two-planed incision closed with a running small nylon suture. At the end of surgery, I would press on the eye to be sure the incision did not leak. Thus it was safe for the patient to move, sneeze, cough, strain, etc. without having the eye collapse as was common with the old incision design. My development of this incision pattern in the early 1970's allowed me to send my patients home

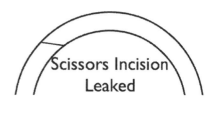

Scissors Incision Leaked

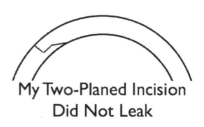

My Two-Planed Incision Did Not Leak

immediately after surgery and allowed for no-stitch surgery later as we began to remove the cataracts through incisions that were only 3.5 to 5 mm. wide. I described this incision in my book A Primer of Cataract and IOL Surgery in 1981.

Intraocular Lenses

Throughout most of the 1970's, people were required to wear very thick cataract glasses after cataract surgery. These glasses made things look 30% too close and 30% too large. Thus they were very disorienting.

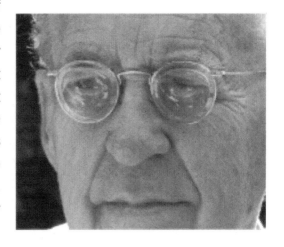

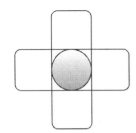 In 1973, Dr. Norman Jaffe came to Dallas and lectured about the small lenses he was placing in eyes after cataract surgery. They were called the "Copeland Lenses" and they were shaped like a cross. They fit into the pupil with two of the supports in front of the iris and two behind. I studied with Dr. Jaffe and began using these lenses. There were only a handful of surgeons using intraocular lenses at this point. In fact, I got fired from my teaching position at the medical school because my chief said, "Anyone so stupid as to put intraocular lenses in eyes has no business teaching residents!" Now it is malpractice not to use them---go figure.

One of the problems with the Copeland lens was that the iris rubbed on it causing chronic inflammation. I began to hear of European surgeons using a different approach. Instead of using solid haptics (support members), they were using 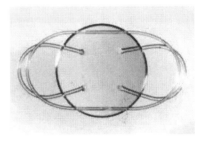 nylon loops to hold the lens in the pupil. Also, the British were using a solid lens placed into the angle where the cornea meets the iris to hold the lens in place. I went to Belgium to study with Cornelius Binkhorst, MD and to Holland to study with Jan Binkhorst, MD in June, 1974.

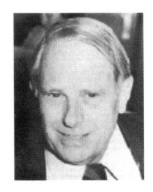

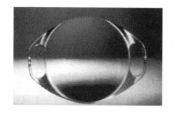

As I was returning home from Holland, I stopped in London. I had made an appointment to see Peter Choyce, MD. Choyce was the resident that assisted when Harold Ridley, MD had

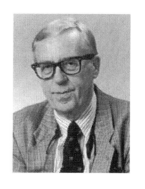

placed the first intraocular lens in an eye on June 28, 1949. (Note: Peter Choyce told me that the first lens was placed on June 28th. I remember that because June 28th is my birthday. Harold Ridley and his surgical nurse (Mrs. Doreen Ogg) both described the first implantation date as being on 29th November 1949, and when in 1999 Ridley was asked whether the IOL's 50th anniversary should be in November 1999 or February 2000 he chose November and attended the celebratory banquet organized by Rayner Optical.)

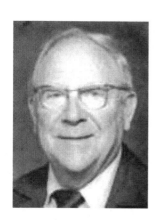

Peter Choyce was in conflict with Sir Stewart Duke-Elder, MD who controlled Moorfields Hospital where he trained. Because he insisted on using intraocular lenses, he was "banished" to a small facility at Southend-on-Sea, about 45 miles east of London. I was tired from my trip to Belgium and Holland and didn't really know how to navigate transportation in the UK. (Remember I am from a town of 328 people and I had never seen an elevator until I went to college.) I started to go back to bed and cancel my appointment with Choyce.

However, I felt that would not be polite so I made myself get up and keep the appointment. That decision would change my life and that of thousands of patients as I would eventually modify what I learned from Choyce that day.

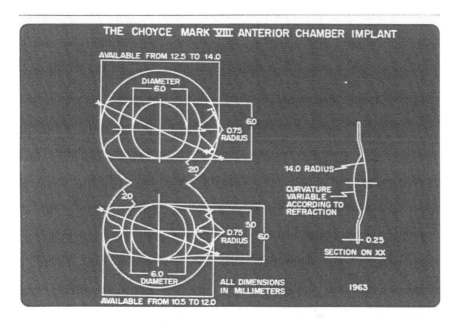

I began to use the Choyce Mark VIII lens in late 1974. I wrote the book A Lens for All Seasons in 1976 to teach surgeons how to use my version of the lens.

I found that most cases of the Choyce Mark VIII lens worked well. However, there were some where the lens caused acute glaucoma because the pupil got stuck on the lens. I changed the lens by making the back of the lens flat. In addition, Choyce's lens moved posterior when the eye was smaller, aggravating the problem. I fixed the distance from the pupil to the back of the lens so it didn't move backward no matter the size of the lens used. This solved the problem.

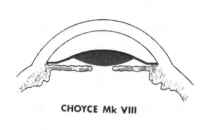

CHOYCE Mk VIII

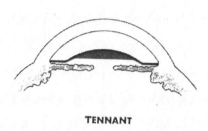

TENNANT

I had been able to get only a few Choyce lenses from Rayner's Optical in London (the only manufacturer). An American manufacturer, Precision Cosmet, agreed to make my modification of the lens. This solved the availability problem and eliminated the glaucoma sometimes seen with Choyce's lens. My lens was called the Tennant Standard Lens. Soon, over 75% of the lenses used in the US were my lens.

The combination of outpatient surgery with intraocular lenses meant that my patients could be too blind to drive and two weeks later, they could have 20/20 vision in each eye and never having experienced any pain or restrictions on their daily activity except not eating the morning of the surgery! What a change from the way I was trained to keep my patient in bed for two weeks after surgery and to try to function with thick glasses. I was able to help make this change in the way ophthalmology was practiced between 1968 and 1976. However, I paid a price much like Peter Choyce did. I was fired from my teaching position at the medical school and banished from my hospital for my efforts. My reward came from my patients, my torment came from my colleagues. Changing paradigms is difficult and often punishing. The concepts in this book will be no different.

Ultraviolet Light Damage

In the early 1970's, I began to recognize the damaging effects of UV light on the eye of the elderly and its role in aging the eye. A pioneer in this area was a professor at Emory University in Atlanta. His laboratory tests confirmed what I was seeing in my patients.

Ultraviolet light is important in the health of the skin and the eye but too much causes burning and damage. In the infant and early childhood, UV light helps to develop vitamin D and the light responses of the eye/retina. That is why it is unwise to put children in sunglasses. However, as the person ages and loses their ability to make nitric oxide to dilate the vessels, the eye becomes more sensitive to UV light. The light damages the structure of the lens of the eye leading to advancing cataracts and it begins to burn the retina that is unable to cool itself due to lack of nitric oxide.

I first studied the results of putting UV filters in glasses after cataract surgery and found there was less macular disease in those that wore UV protecting glasses.

I then worried that the light from my operating microscope would damage the retina during eye surgery. I created UV filters and attached them to one of my microscopes. I proved that I had more macular damage in those operated on with the unfiltered microscope than with the filtered one. This eventually lead to all of the microscope manufacturers adding UV filters to their microscopes and to postoperative glasses having UV filters as well.

I then insisted that all of my intraocular lenses had UV filters built into the lens. Now all intraocular lenses contain these filters.

Anti-prostaglandin Drugs in Ophthalmology
In the 1970's, cataracts were removed including their capsule. This created a space in the eye that allowed the vitreous to move forward. If it was attached to the macula, it would pull on it creating small cysts or a larger cyst or hole. This condition called "cystoid macular edema" or "macular cyst" was a common complication of intracapsular surgery of those days. No one knew how to treat it. Sometimes it went away with time---sometimes there was permanent loss of vision.

Indomethacin is a drug that blocks inflammation. It is in the same family as aspirin but much stronger. It was approved for use in the US in 1965. By the 1970's, it was popular for treating arthritis. I wondered if it would help inflammation in the eye. Taking it orally often caused severe GI symptoms, so I began to mix the contents of the capsule in Tear Drops for the eye. I found it very useful in all sorts of inflammation of the eye including cystoid macular edema. After my reports at medical meetings, the drug companies began to develop this family of eye drops. They are now some of the most widely used eye medications.

Intraocular Lens Manufacture

Harold Ridley noted that fighter pilots that got fragments of the Spitfire aircraft windshield in their eyes tolerated them well if the fragments didn't move, but tolerated them poorly with inflammation, glaucoma and bleeding if the fragments moved in the eye. To make his first lens implant, he contacted the manufacturer of the aircraft windshields and had his lenses made from that same plastic. It was called Perspex CQ.

Not all lenses have been crafted well. Strampelli is said to have made his lenses from a crashed automobile windshield. He is known to have problems with his lenses.

Rayner's Optical made the lenses for Ridley, Choyce, Pearce, etc. They were carefully ground and polished. Precision Cosmet did the same with my lenses being sure the edges were all smooth by a technique called tumble polishing.

One day executives from a company called Surgidev came to my office and wanted to know what was special about my lens. I told them I could tell them but that my lens was patented and that Precision Cosmet had an exclusive right to make them. They told me that if they liked my lens, they would make it and I could sue them. They did indeed copy my lens. However, they used a manufacturing technique called injection molding. A mold is made and then plastic is injected into the mold. This always leaves a tag of plastic where the plastic was injected into the mold. In addition, the quality of the edges is determined by how the mold was made. If the mold has sharp corners (difficult not to have in a mold), the lenses will have sharp edges. However, it is a less expensive way to make lenses. Unfortunately, these sharp edges cut the iris as it moves across the supporting haptics of the lens. This leads to inflammation (uveitis), glaucoma, and bleeding (hyphema). This became known as the "UGH" syndrome. This cutting of corners in manufacturing lead to a bad reputation for all anterior chamber supported lenses and to surgeons abandoning them. No one ever reported a single case of the UGH syndrome with my lenses, but surgeons never recognized that hospitals/surgicenters buying these cheap, imitation lenses were destroying eyes and the reputation of great lenses. By the time the courts heard our case, they was no longer a market for our lenses.

Excimer Laser Surgery
A dream of most that wear glasses is to see without them. A Russian ophthalmologist, Svyatoslav Nikolayevich Fyodorov, MD, treated a 16 year old boy that cut his eye with a piece of glass. The boy had been quite near-sighted before the injury. Afterwards, his near-sightedness was gone. Fyodorov decided to purposely do this by making surgical

incisions in the cornea. This became known as "Radial Keratotomy". Leo Bores, MD saw Fyodorov perform this and brought the technique to the US. Others soon followed. There were problems with the procedure including becoming far-sighted over time as the cornea weakened and bulged.

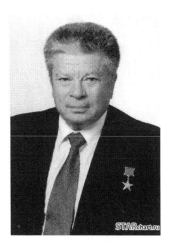

Three researchers at the IBM's Thomas J. Watson Research Center in Yorktown, New York—Samuel Blum, Rangaswamy Srinivasan and James J. Wynne—had been exploring new ways to use the excimer laser that had been recently acquired by their laser physics and chemistry group. They wondered what it would do on animal tissue, so they tried it on left-over Thanksgiving turkey on November 26, 1981. They found it would very precisely cut away microns of tissue.

Steven Trokel, MD of Columbia University in New York was writing a new book about the use of lasers in ophthalmology. He ran across some writings about the new excimer laser and soon was working with Srinivasan at IBM to test it on corneas. This eventually became the procedure of choice for changing the need for glasses.

In 1987, Marguerite McDonald, MD performed the first human treatment of near-sightedness with the excimer laser. After completing the Phase I FDA study on blind eyes and the Phase II FDA study on partially-sighted eyes, Phase III was opened to other researchers. I was one of twelve selected for this study. I personally performed 80% of the study with the other eleven researchers doing 20%. I did about 1000 cases in the US and about 2000 cases abroad.

Initially, we treated the eyes by removing the epithelial lining of the eye with a scalpel and then reshaping the structural part of the cornea with the excimer laser. This was called "Photo-refractive Keratectomy" or "PRK". Later a procedure called "Laser-Assisted Sub-Epithelial Keratectomy (or Laser Epithelial Keratomileusis) (LASEK or LASIK) was developed in which a flap of the cornea was lifted and the cornea was reshaped under the flap. This allowed for faster healing but could be associated with complications from making the flap.

I inhaled viruses while doing this research. I developed encephalitis and a bleeding disorder from this work. (A root canal tooth dropped my voltage allowing me to be susceptible to these infections). This lead to my having to stop working less than two months before the research caused the FDA to approve the laser for general usage.

This book is the result of my having to figure out how to get myself well from the disabling effects of my research efforts to eliminate the need for glasses for the millions that have benefited from the work.

Expulsive Hemorrhage During Surgery

One thing every eye surgeon fears is an expulsive hemorrhage during surgery. This means that when you make an incision in the eye, a blood vessel inside the eye ruptures causing hemorrhage into the eye. This causes the contents of the eye to suddenly be expelled out of the eye resulting in blindness.

Performing thousands of eye surgeries over the course of 30 years, I only lost a few eyes, mostly due to infection. However, I will always remember one particular lady. She was in her late 80's and had lost the vision in one eye before she came to see me. The cataract in her remaining eye was severe with only hand motion vision. I began a routine surgery I thought. However, as soon as I made the incision, she had an expulsive hemorrhage and her retina was on her cheek. I had no training that had taught me how to prevent this. I was devastated! Now she was totally blind.

I began to consider how I could have prevented this. One has no control over fragile and brittle blood vessels. However, I could always have a "seat belt" to quickly close the incision. I began to always put strong sutures into the wound before I actually entered the eye interior. This way I could quickly block the exit of the critical eye structures. Next, I needed a way to deal with the hemorrhage itself. Without being able to get the blood out of the eye, the pressure would build up and occlude the circulation to the retina. I found that I could make four tiny incisions about five mm. behind where the cornea meets the sclera. I would then cauterize the lips of these incision so they would stay open like a fish mouth. If the eye was bleeding, I could gently press a spatula onto the muscle (ciliary body) under these incisions and whatever blood was in the eye would come out of these incisions. If the eye was simply too hard from pressure, I could stick a very small needle through this muscle into the center of the eye and safely withdraw 0.1 cc of fluid. This would always lower the pressure. I would sit there for 5-10 minutes waiting for the bleeding to stop. I could then safely continue the surgery. After developing this technique, I never again lost an eye although I had to deal with bleeding several times.

Dropped Nucleus

Another event that puts fear into the heart of an eye surgeon is to have the lens of the eye (nucleus) drop into the back of the eye. Surgeons that normally operate on the front of the eye for cataract and corneal surgery are not trained what to do when this happens. They are trained to close up the eye and send the patient to a retinal surgeon to remove the dropped lens. This means a second surgery and a delay that causes a considerable amount of inflammation of the retina.

It is easier to remove the dropped lens through the front of the eye than through the sclera (where I made the incisions I showed in the previous image). However, the problem is the same as getting your hook trapped in weeds while you are fishing. You are trying to pull the hook upward and the weeds prevent you from doing so.

When you reach down into the vitreous (center of the eye) to attempt to pull the nucleus out, it gets snagged on the vitreous floating on

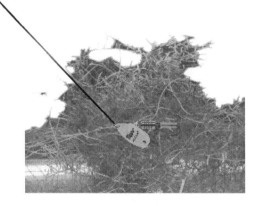

188

top of the fluid in the eye. This pulls it off your instrument and it drops back into the eye again.

What one needs to do is make a hole in the center of the

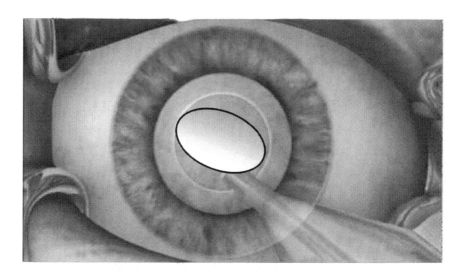

weeds (vitreous) so you can pull the nucleus out without difficulty. This is done with a tool called a vitrector. One then inserts the Phako tool that is used to pulverize the nucleus down into the center of the eye. Pulsing it causes the nucleus up to its tip where it can be captured and easily pulled from the eye. One can then continue with placing the intraocular lens and the day after surgery, the vision is great just as if nothing complicated the surgery!

I have attempted to share with you some of the things I contributed to ophthalmology. I don't do this for self-aggrandizement. However, many would dismiss what I am going to share with you in the rest of the book if you didn't know that I have already solved many problems of curing eye diseases and surgical problems in the past.

Using what I learned in the efforts to get myself well, I have figured out how to reverse macular degeneration, optic neuritis, glaucoma, corneal dystrophy, and cataracts. These are the major causes of blindness. The cases that have progressed to scarring do not respond, but by changing their paradigm, ophthalmologists and patients will be able to get vision back if treated early.

9 Cataracts

The human eye has some similarities to a camera. There is a lens system at the front and a film at the back where the image is focused.

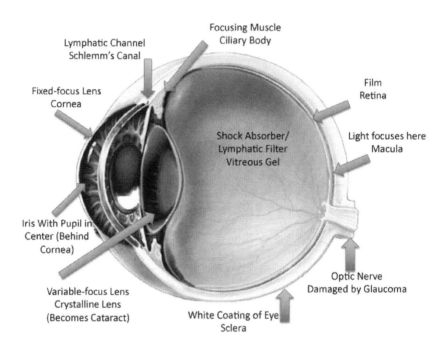

The front of the eye has a clear window called the cornea. It serves as a fixed-focus lens. Behind this fixed-focus lens is a diaphragm in the center of a muscle called the iris. The iris is the colored part of the eye that you see when you look at someone. You don't see the clear cornea that is in front of it. Since the muscle can move, it can make the hole in the center of it larger or smaller to let more or less light into the eye. This hole is called the pupil.

Just behind the pupil is the variable-focus lens. It is called the crystalline lens. It is suspended from a circular muscle called the ciliary body. As this muscle adjusts the tension on the crystalline lens, it changes shape and thus changes its power. This allows it to focus the image on the retina (macula) as the image moves closer to the eye or farther away. It is this lens that keeps things in focus as you pull something closer to you to read.

In a perfect eye, the power of the fixed-focus cornea plus the power of the variable-focus crystalline lens when it is at rest will be perfect to focus the image of a distant object onto the macula at the center of the retina. Then as you pull the image closer to you, the variable-focus crystalline lens adds more power so the image will stay in focus.

As you get to be about forty years old, the crystalline lens becomes too stiff to add enough power to keep near objects in focus so you have to start wearing reading glasses.

When the length of the eye matches the power of the lens system, the eye is normal. When the length of the eye is too long for the power of the lens system, the image focuses in front of the retina. Thus everything is blurry unless you pull the object closer to your face. Doing so pushes the image back to the retina so it becomes in focus. To see at distance, you must wear glasses that push the image back onto the retina.

When the length of the eye is too short for the power of the

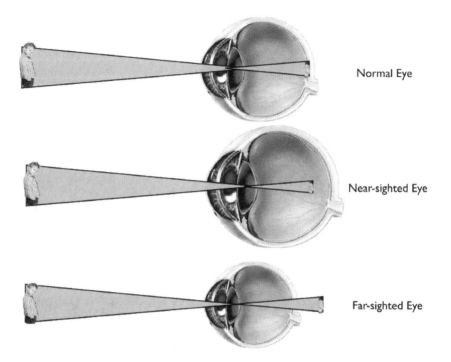

Normal Eye

Near-sighted Eye

Far-sighted Eye

lens system, the image is focused behind the eye. Thus it is also blurry. The only way you can make it clear is to add focusing power. Sometimes the eye is young enough to add enough focusing power with the variable focus lens. However, over time, the power of the variable-focus crystalline lens becomes inadequate to keep you in focus and thus you need glasses for distance as well as reading.

Over time, the variable-focus crystalline lens of the eye becomes hazy and then opaque. This is called a **cataract.**

The crystalline lens is made mostly of water and protein. Specific proteins within the lens are responsible for keeping

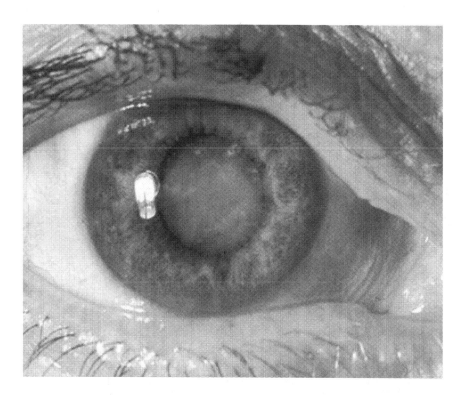

it clear. Over many years, the structures of these lens proteins are altered, leading to a gradual clouding of the lens. Causes of cataracts include:

1. Ultraviolet light exposure (not wearing sunglasses)
2. Infrared light: seen in welders and glass blowers
3. Nutritional deficiencies
    a. Vitamin C
    b. Vitamin E
    c. Carotenoids: lutein, zeaxanthin, astaxanthin
4. Diabetes
5. Smoking
6. Using steroid medications orally or topically
7. Glaucoma medications
8. Dental infections
9. Statin drugs (cholesterol lowering drugs)
10. Phenothiazine drugs (like Thorazine and Compazine)

11. Trauma
12. Uveitis (inflammation in the eye)
13. Birth defect
14. Eye surgery (touching the lens during surgery)

However, the main cause of cataracts is lipid peroxidation of the epithelial layer of the lens. Lipid peroxidation refers to the oxidative degradation (damage by electron stealers) of lipids. It is the process in which free radicals "steal" electrons from the lipids in cell membranes, resulting in cell damage. This process proceeds by a free radical chain reaction mechanism. It most often affects polyunsaturated fatty acids, because they contain multiple double bonds in between which lie methylene -CH2- groups that possess especially reactive hydrogens (strong electron stealers). wikipedia

A primary way the body deals with protecting double bonds is with iodine. As you will recall, almost everyone in the US is iodine deficient.

Age-related cataract is responsible for 48% of world blindness, which represents about 18 million people, according to the World Health Organization (WHO). In many countries surgical services are inadequate, and cataracts remain the leading cause of blindness.

Age Range	Incidence of Cataracts in US
52-64	42%
65-74	60%
75-85	91%

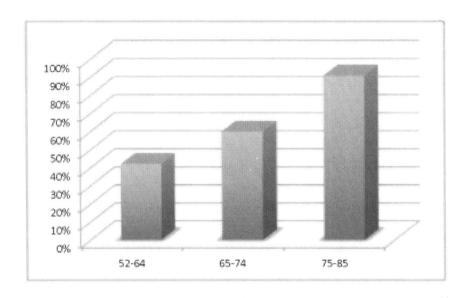

The increase in ultraviolet radiation resulting from depletion of the ozone layer is expected to increase the incidence of cataracts. [Wikipedia]

Reversing Cataracts

Our ability to reverse damaged cells in the human body with voltage, nutrition, correcting cellular software, and removal of toxins is primarily dependent upon how much scarring is present. Once cells become scar tissue, it is much harder to correct because regeneration is harder than simply making new cells. Regeneration implies that you have created new stem cells that are able to form natural cells plus the ability to replace scar tissue with normal cells. Regeneration therefore means that you must turn normal cells back into stem cells and then have them become the type of cell you wish to replace. Compare that with simply "charging up" a sluggish cell and allowing it to make a new copy of itself.

The medical rule for removing cataracts used to be that you should have surgery to remove a cataract whenever the amount of vision you have left is inadequate to do the things you need to do. A fifty year old that must drive to work and read every day needs better vision to do their daily task than a ninety year old that moves from bed to couch to dinner table and back every day and the most challenging thing they do with their vision is watching TV.

However, the insurance companies, particularly Medicare, changed the guidelines. They say that your vision must be 20/50 or worse to qualify for them to pay for your surgery. (20/50 means that you have to be 20 feet from something that a normal eye can see from 50 feet. It is also the vision necessary to read a newspaper.)

It turns out that the 20/50 level is about the amount of haziness of the crystalline lens that can be reversed with correcting the voltage, nutrition, software and toxins that affect the eye. If your vision is 20/50 or better due to a cataract, it can often be made better. However, if the vision is 20/50 or worse, you will likely have to have the cataract removed surgically.

We have discussed in the chapters on voltage and the BioModulator how we can measure and correct the voltage in the eye.

To provide the amino acids necessary to make new cells, we must correct the function of your stomach acid. This is because stomach acid is required to turn the proteins you eat into the amino acids you need to make new cells. Making stomach acid requires iodine, zinc, and vitamin B1. To adsorb zinc requires stomach acid. Thus you must take Betaine or apple cider vinegar with your zinc so it will be absorbed.

To get the amino acids and other vitamins and minerals into cells requires fulvic acid. We have developed a proprietary blend of fulvic acid with the nutrients needed to nourish cells called Raw Materials.

We have also developed blends of essential oils that can help correct the software (signals from DNA to the proteins of cells) so that they work correctly.

You must also identify any teeth that have infections (cavities, infections under crowns, or root canals/infection in bone) that are connected to the eyes via the acupuncture system that are sending toxins to the eyes. These infections must be removed.

It is also important to help the body remove toxins by supporting the detoxification organs of the body including the liver/gall bladder system, kidneys, large intestine and skin.

Identifying what needs to be done in each person requires an in-office evaluation and treatments for 1-2 weeks. However, the healing process of making new cells goes on for several weeks afterward as the body receives the nutrients necessary to make new cells and as you eliminate the toxins that damage new and old cells alike.

10 Macular Degeneration

Macular Degeneration

The retina contains two types of receptors. Rods are designed to perceive whether it is light or dark and movement. Cones are designed to detect color and fine detail. Thus it is our cones that allow us to read and see colors. The cones are concentrated in the center of the retina where the light focuses. This is called the macula.

A common problem is a degeneration of the cones in the macula so that we have a gradual loss of vision. We never go blind in the sense that the lights go out but we lose our ability to see colors, read, see road signs, distinguish one face from another, etc. This is called macular degeneration.

Up until about 15-20 years ago, it was called "senile macular degeneration". Over time, we began to see it in younger and younger people and the name morphed into "age-related macular degeneration" or ARMD.

Early signs of macular degeneration are scars called "drusen". These are yellow waxy balls that resemble

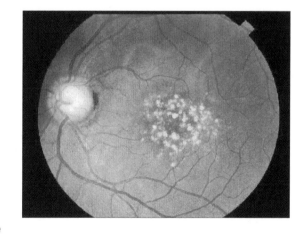

plaques inside arteries in atherosclerosis. As more cones degenerate, more drusen form. This is called "dry" macular degeneration. Over time, new blood vessels begin to grow into the damaged area in the same way as new blood vessels grow into scarred heart tissue after a heart attack. However, where this is helpful in the heart, these new blood vessels in the eye damage vision and may even bleed into the macula. This is called "wet" macular degeneration.

Wet macular degeneration may be treated with a laser to seal leaky vessels, but the laser often causes additional damage to the retina. In addition, the vessels almost always grow back. Now it is popular to inject a drug into the eye that tends to constrict these new blood vessels. However, the drugs do not address the reason that the vessels are growing in the first place.

Current treatments for macular degeneration are discussed in the paper Age-related Macular Degeneration Review of Current Treatments; Preeti R Poley; William M Stapleton; Fang Qui; Michael L Mulhern; David D Ingvoldstad; Eyal Margalit; Expert Rev Ophthalmol. 2011;6 (2):195-201.

Dry Macular Degeneration: The Age-Related Eye Disease Study (AREDS) found that the natural history of progression to advanced macular degeneration was:

Amount of AMD at Start	Risk of Progression in Five Years
None	0.4%
Early MAD	1.3%

Amount of AMD at Start	Risk of Progression in Five Years
Intermediate AMD	18%
Advanced AMD	43%

The AREDS2 Study is looking at whether anti-oxidants like lutein, zeaxanthin and omega-3 fats are useful in treating macular degeneration.

Wet Macular Degeneration:

The Macular Photocoagulation Study demonstrated that focal laser photocoagulation of new blood vessels in the macular area reduced the risk of severe vision loss, but also demonstrated an approximate 50% recurrence rate of new blood vessels.

The Treatment of Age-Related Macular Degeneration by injection of a photosensitive material and then using a laser to activate the material found that 47% of patients with predominantly classic lesions lost vision (three or more lines) when treated with photodynamic therapy (PDT), versus 62% in the placebo group. The Verteporfin in Photodynamic Therapy (VIP) trial demonstrated that 55% of patients with occult lesions experienced vision loss when treated with PDT compared with 68% in placebo.

In the ANCHOR AND MARINA trials, the drug ranibizumab (Lucentis) was shown to improve vision when compared with placebo injections.

Bevacizumab (Avastin) is being used in other countries but not the US.

Neither ranibizumab (Lucentis) nor bevacizumab (Avastin) have had any long-term studies for safety and efficacy!

In May 2011, a one year study was released comparing ranibizumab (Lucentis) with bevacizumab (Avastin) in wet macular degeneration. The results were equal even though ranibizumab (Lucentis) costs about $2000 per injection and bevacizumab (Avastin) costs about $50 per injection. Bevacizumab (Avastin) is approved in the US as a cancer drug but not for macular degeneration. However, since the same company owns both drugs, they do not appear to be motivated to get the less expensive drug approved for macular degeneration.

A troubling aspect of either drug is the side effects. The rates of death, myocardial infarction and stroke were similar in the 2 groups, but a higher proportion of bevacizumab (Avastin) patients (24.1%) had "serious systemic adverse events (primarily hospitalization)" compared to the ranibizumab (Lucentis) group (19%). It is troubling that so many that receive this therapy have serious side effects. It is not clear to me if all patients know that there is a 20-25% chance they will end up in the hospital after having this treatment!

I am now going to discuss methods not described in the above review of current therapies. The traditional treatment of dry macular degeneration with anti-oxidants is only minimally successful in stopping the progression of macular degeneration and rarely reverses it. I will discuss how to do both.

Retinal Function

Most theories and research about retinal function have followed the Newtonian-Reductionism paradigm. Efforts continue to explain retinal function purely on a chemical basis. Most theories consider that chemical reactions in certain cells somehow create voltage that is passed along the nerve fibers of the optic nerve and on to the brain. The purpose of this chapter is to suggest a different paradigm

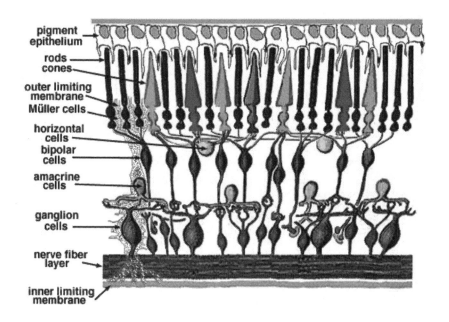

based on electronic theory.

The retina is composed of three basic layers:
1. Photoreceptors (rods and cones)

2. Bipolar layer (connects photoreceptors to ganglion layer)
3. Ganglion cell layer (part of the optic nerve) [9]

Light passes through the transparent retina and strikes the opaque pigment epithelium. As it passes through the photoreceptors, light that is in phase with any given receptor is recognized by that receptor because the receptor is an antenna tuned to that frequency by its resonating circuitry.

A look at the microanatomy reveals that rods and cones are shaped just like the light-reception antenna of insects and contain resonating circuits. [10] [11] [12]

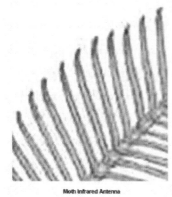

Moth Infrared Antenna

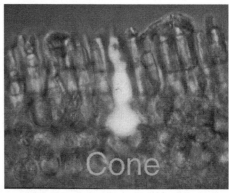

Cone

As can be seen in this electron photomicrograph, the photoreceptors are shaped like insect and commercial radio/TV antennas. Inside, they contain a coil structure similar to a drill auger. This structure is the coil portion of a Tesla Impedance/Capacitance (LC) circuit. The pedicle contains parallel bars that create the capacitor. Thus we have a typical LC circuit used to tune antennas throughout

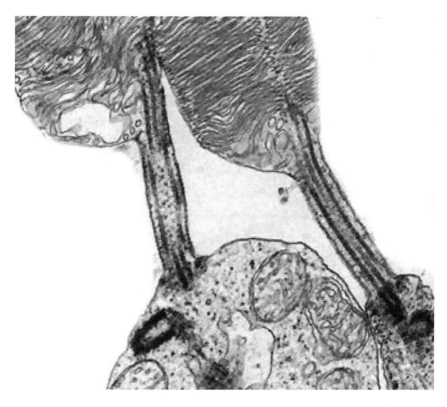

electronics and biological systems.

The basic lengths of the antennas (photoreceptors) are approximate to their intended light frequency. Thus rods are more tuned to the infrared light that constantly surrounds the earth day and night. Since infrared/red light is a longer wavelength than visible light, it would require a longer antenna to receive that wavelength. Cones receive visible light and thus would require an antenna shorter than the infrared/red light. We see that they are indeed anatomically shorter than rods.

The energy of the light that resonates in photoreceptors is stored until it reaches critical storage capacity. It is then discharged. The electrons then pass into the bipolar cell region. The bipolar cells function like tubes or transistors in an electronic circuit. They control the flow of electrons according to their design and create an image. These images in digital format are passed to the brain via the ganglion cell layer/optic nerve fibers.

A critical issue in this electronic circuit and any other is operating voltage. Just as your radio won't function without a power source, neither will your retina. In the body, electrons are most efficiently transferred from place to place by "fibrous wires" more commonly known as fascia and glial cells. In the retina, the voltage is transmitted across the retina by glial cells known as Muller cells. These transmit electrons to all layers of the retina. Muller fibers can receive voltage in an ionic transfer from the connections of the choroid and via light via the inner limiting membrane.

"Muller (radial glial) cells span the entire thickness of the retina, and contact and ensheath every type of neuronal cell body and process. This morphological relationship is reflected by a multitude of functional interactions between retinal neurons and Muller cells, including extracellular ion homeostasis and glutamate recycling by Muller cells. **Virtually every disease of the retina is associated with a reactive Muller cell gliosis. (scarring)"** [13]

One of the causes of damage to these cells is that free radicals (electron stealers) and singlet oxygen (an electron

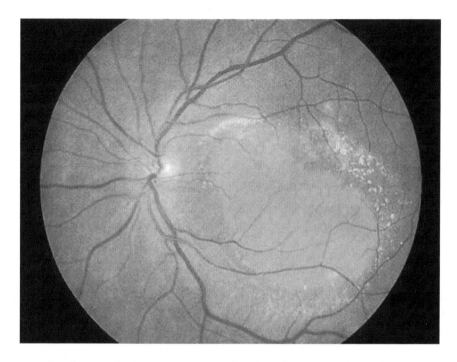

stealer form of oxygen created by light) oxidize fatty acids in your retina, compromising your retinal cell membranes and causing damage.

As Björn Nordenstrom [4], Robert Becker [5] and others have shown, chronic disease is associated with a loss of voltage. Loss of the Muller cells that carry voltage to the entire retina would imply that the retina would lose voltage and thus its ability to function normally.

Summary: In electronics, components like capacitors, coils, resistors, circuit connectors, etc. are made from various materials. In the human, these same components exist, but they are made from a combination of proteins, fats, and rarely, carbohydrates. Focus has been on changes within these proteins, fats and carbohydrates during the process of vision rather than on the electronic circuitry. One can more easily understand dysfunctional electronic devices by measuring their quantum physics attributes than by considering the chemical reactions inside the transistors, capacitors, etc. So it is with vision.

The photoreceptors are antennae containing LC circuits. These LC circuits are connected to bipolar cells that act as transistors controlling and processing the digital imagery transmitted to the ganglion cells and thus to the brain. Power is supplied to these circuits via the Muller cells. They are connected to other sources of ongoing power.

Restoration of degenerations of the retina must certainly require restoration of the voltage to the retina so it can, like other electronic circuits, restore its function.

In 2003, I noticed that sometimes macular degeneration improved when we were treating patients with the Russian SCENAR. I decided to focus on how predictable this might be. I knew that the Russians that manufactured the SCENAR did not have the money to fund a study. Normally, manufacturers fund studies that prove the efficacy of their products. Thus it fell to me to attempt to help people with this technology. Remember that I had been sick and bankrupt for about seven years, so my resources were scant as well. I had two options: to simply treat people off-label and see the results or set up a pilot study using published FDA guidelines. I decided to do the latter.

The FDA publishes their guidelines for studies in the Federal Register. I printed them out and then created the pilot study to fulfill their requirements including creating an

Investigational Review Board to supervise the study. I then found patients and treated them for free.

Then an unusual thing happened. A woman came to my office with a friend from her church. They said that the church was going to pay for her exam. She complained of fibromyalgia. I examined her and made recommendations for her care. When she went to the desk to check out, she told my receptionist that her exam was free. When asked why, she said that we were treating macular degeneration free. She was told that was true but she did not have macular degeneration and that there would be a fee for her exam. The friend from church paid the fee.

A few days later she called the office and insisted that we refund her fee because she was not satisfied with her exam. We told her that we would refund the fee but that it must be returned to the church that paid it instead of giving the money to her. She was furious that we would not give her the money and told us that she was going to report us to the FDA. She did. This caused the FDA to come to my office to look at our study.

The FDA found deficiencies that were not part of their published requirements. For example, they found us deficient for not having a study coordinator when the requirements in the Federal Register do not require a study coordinator. They found us non-compliant because we had a signature line on the front of the Informed Consent instead of the last page of the consent. They found us non-compliant because a family member that is an MD was on the Investigational Review Board in spite of the Federal

Register stating this was acceptable. We did have a
legitimate problem in that two of the patient charts
disappeared. I have no idea whether the patients took them
home or if my staff misfiled them. They were never found.

DEPARTMENT OF HEALTH & HUMAN SERVICES   Public Health Service

_____

Food and Drug Administration
9200 Corporate Boulevard
Rockville, Maryland 20850

AUG 3 1 2007

Jerald E. Tennant, MD
Synergy Medical Group
5601 North MacArthur Blvd., Suite 200
Irving, TX 75038

Dear Dr. Tennant:

The purpose of this letter is to inform you that the Food and Drug Administration (FDA)
inspection conducted at your clinical site during the period of July 12 through 13, 2007,
revealed no significant concerns. As a result, no response is necessary at this time.

The inspection was conducted by an investigator from FDA's Dallas District Office and
covered your activities as a clinical investigator in the study entitled *SCENAR
Electromagnetic Therapy for Treatment of Macular Degeneration.* The SCENAR is a
device as defined in Section 201(h) of the Federal Food, Drug, and Cosmetic Act (the
Act).

We appreciate the courtesy and cooperation extended to the FDA investigator during the
inspection and subsequent closeout discussion. You may find information concerning the
device Bioresearch Monitoring program at our Internet homepage,
http://www.fda.gov/cdrh/comp/bimo.html. Valuable links to related information are also
included at this site.

If you have any questions, please contact the BIMO reviewer, Cynthia A. Harris, MS,
RN, at (240) 276-0125, or at cynthia.harris@fda.hhs.gov.

Sincerely yours,

Doreen M. Kezer, MSN
Chief, Special Investigations Branch
Division of Bioresearch Monitoring
Office of Compliance
Center for Devices and Radiological Health

This resulted in the FDA issuing me a Warning Letter
outlining their complaints. They returned for a follow-up and

issued a letter on August 31, 2007 stating that we were in compliance and that no further action was indicated.

What we found was that all the cases that still had 20/70 vision or better got significant improvement in their vision. Those that were worse than 20/70 did not get back to reading vision (20/50) but stabilized. Those that did not show improvement were primarily those with scarring like seen in this image. We did not continue the study with the Russian SCENAR. We could barely afford the pilot study and the expense created by the FDA put it beyond our capabilities.

Since that time, we have learned better ways to treat macular degeneration. I developed the BioModulator. We have developed better frequency sets in the Tennant BioModulator that are more efficient at transferring voltage to the cell membranes. Cells run at -20 to -25 millivolts (pH of 7.35 to 7.45) and you need -50 millivolts to make new cells. Using the BioModulator off-label, we found that we can restore the voltage to the retina to heal the macular degeneration by making new cells.

The brain and retina are made from fat. The brain is 50% cholesterol by weight. Taking statin drugs has no significant benefit in preventing heart attacks (only one person out of 2,000 benefits from lowering cholesterol as far as heart attacks is concerned) but can influence the ability of the brain/eye to heal.

The ratio of omega-3 to omega-6 fats is important. We get plenty of omega-6 fats in our diet, but most are deficient in omega-3 fats. They must be supplemented if you don't eat lots of fish, nuts, and other sources of omega-3 fats.

Another problem is the gall bladder and bile system. You can't absorb fats if you don't have a gall bladder to store bile. If you want to have fat available to rebuild your brain/eyes, you will need to take bile with each meal to absorb the fats you need to rebuild your cells.

In oriental medicine, it is taught that the liver meridian is the primary concern for the eyes. However, we have found that the acupuncture meridian that relates most to retinal problems is the spleen meridian. Most that have macular degeneration will have decreased voltage in the spleen meridian and many will have an infected tooth in this meridian. An infected tooth puts out poisons called thio-ethers and glio-toxins. This is often the driving force behind macular degeneration and particularly pre-macular membranes. I have yet to see a pre-macular membrane that was not associated with a dental infection in the spleen meridian. To permanently overcome this problem the dental infection must be resolved including pulling any root canal teeth in the meridians that serve the eyes. These include triple burner, liver and bladder meridians.

Circulation in the body is controlled by nitric oxide. It is the master hormone in the body and also dilates almost everything that needs to be dilated like blood vessels, bronchioles, and lymphatics. Thus it is important to correct nitric oxide. This can be accomplished with nutrients providing you also correct stomach acid. Stomach acid is required to break proteins down into amino acids including those needed to make nitric oxide. I discuss this in the chapter on Nitric Oxide.

It is also necessary to restore the vitamins and minerals to the retinal cells. This is best accomplished with natural products instead of vitamins manufactured from petroleum. Phytoplankton is the primary source from the ocean and humic is the primary source from the land.

How We Reverse Macular Degeneration

We ask people with macular degeneration to set aside a week to begin to correct it. They come to our clinic twice a day for five days. We determine the state of the eye and current vision. We look for dental infections that may be contributing to decreased vision. We test for nitric oxide levels and mineral deficiencies. We then begin the process of restoring voltage with the BioModulator and its attachments. The eyes are treated for about 10-15 minutes each, twice a day.

Although the amount of scarring present will determine your result, in most cases those with vision of 20/70 or better will be 20/30 or better at the end of the five days. Often the vision continues to improve even after the five days of treatment as the nutrients and correction of nitric oxide are achieved. It generally takes about three months to correct these issues. Maintenance therapy will likely be needed.

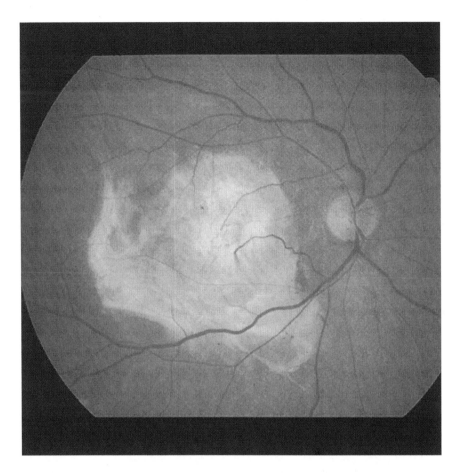

If there is an infected tooth in the meridians to the eyes, your improvement will be diminished until the infection is removed by your dentist. Remember that root canal teeth are dead tissue and are always infected. The only way to correct them is to remove them.

Many studies have shown that using antioxidants (electron donors) help macular degeneration. Two significant ones are astaxanthin and ubiquinol.

11 Glaucoma

The word "glaucoma" implies that the pressure inside the eye is high enough to cause damage to the optic nerve that runs from the retina of the eye to the brain. This damage causes you to lose your ability to see.

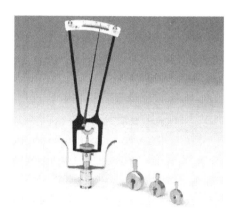

There have been many things developed to measure the pressure inside the eye. The first was to simply use your fingers to see if the eye feels abnormally hard. Obviously this is very subjective and cannot identify small, but significant, increases in pressure. Next was a device called the Schiotz tonometer. This device has a piston that moves up and down inside a shaft that has a curved end to fit onto the cornea (front clear part of the eye). How deep the piston will indent the eye is determined by three factors:

1. The pressure inside the eye
2. The weight of the piston
3. The stiffness of the tissue

One can increase the weight of the piston by adding a washer of known weight to it. This is only necessary if the eye pressure is very high.

The Schiotz tonometer was used for many years as the standard method for measuring eye pressure and is still a very economical method of doing so.

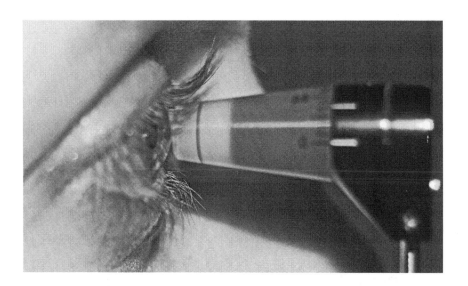

The applanation tonometer was the next device invented for measuring pressure. The basic concept is that one presses a flat plate of known diameter against the cornea of the eye until the cornea touches exactly all of the flat plate. One can determine the pressure necessary to cause the eye to flatten exactly this amount and convert that pressure into the pressure of the eye. Obviously the higher the pressure in the eye, the more pressure it will take to flatten it to a known amount. The applanation tonometer is usually attached to the eye microscope (known as a slit lamp) so the doctor/ nurse can view down the center of the tonometer head to see when the exact flattening occurs.

For many years the applanation tonometer was the "gold standard" for measuring eye pressure. It does require the skill of someone that can effectively use the eye microscope. This encouraged the use of a device that did not require that skill and could thus be performed by someone not able to use the microscope. In addition, both the Schiotz tonometer and the applanation tonometer require the use of an anesthetic drop to numb the eye to perform the test. Many years ago, optometrists were not licensed to use these medications, so there was a stimulus to find another way to measure eye pressures. This led to the development of the "puff tonometer". This involves blowing a puff of air of known quantity and intensity at the cornea. The distortion caused by this puff of air changes the reflection of light from the cornea. This distortion can be measured and converted to an estimate of the eye pressure. This device is convenient for having a staff member measure the pressure, but it is generally hated by patients because of the startle that occurs even when you know the blast of air into your eye is coming.

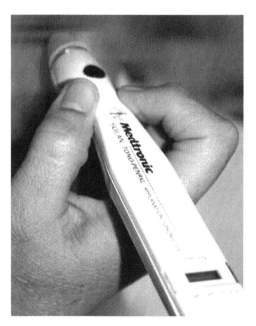

In the 1990's, a miniaturized and digitized version of the Schiotz tonometer was developed. It is called the Tonopen. One can simply "peck" at the cornea with this device and it will give you the pressure. One advantage is that one can measure in the periphery of the cornea away from where Lasik is performed. Measuring over the site of Lasik surgery with a Schiotz, applanation tonometer, or puff tonometer gives abnormally low readings. Since so many people have had Lasik surgery, the Tonopen has become widely used.

You may experience any of these methods of measuring pressure when you visit your eye doctor.

There are several things that can give erroneous readings:
1. Pressure from the squeezing of your eyelids while the pressure is being taken.
2. Pressure from the fingers of the examiner.
3. Change in the thickness of the cornea.
4. Change in the elasticity of the sclera (white covering of the eye).
5. Holding your breath while taking the pressure.

How Does An Increased Pressure Damage the Eye?

The eye is a part of the nervous system. As such, it has a high demand for voltage, oxygen, and glucose. All cells in the body are designed to run on fat as their primary fuel except for neurons. They are designed to run on glucose. A normal liver can store about 1 1/2 hours of glucose for the nervous system and then it must be replenished if the nervous system is to run correctly. As fuel (glucose) runs low, it is often vision symptoms that you notice first as your nervous system begins to malfunction.

The way that glucose and oxygen get to the eyes is by way of the vascular system. If your circulation is inadequate, the nervous system begins to malfunction and eventually the neurons die.

The ability of the cardiovascular system and the respiratory system to bring blood and oxygen to the eyes is a careful balance of both systems. Your heart must beat adequately to push the blood to the head and lungs. You must have enough hemoglobin in your blood to carry oxygen to the eyes. Your lungs must be able to move air in and out to provide oxygen to the blood so it can be distributed throughout the body.

A great problem in Western Medicine is that doctors forget that the body is a SYSTEM. Heart doctors want the blood pressure as low as they can get it. The reason is that the lower the blood pressure, the less work is placed on the heart. They forget that it takes adequate pressure to push blood uphill to the brain and eyes. Heart doctors and family practitioners/internists forget we have a brain and eyes. Eye doctors forget we have a heart and often don't check blood pressure to see if it is adequate to serve the needs of the eyes. Both heart doctors and eye doctors tend to ignore the fact that the liver is the "fuel tank" for the brain and the eyes.

Almost everyone forgets that neurons in the eyes replace themselves every couple of days. Since they are made from fat, there needs to be a constant supply of fat to be able to make new cells. If you are on a low fat diet, it is hard to maintain your brain, eyes, and nervous system.

You cannot absorb the fat you eat if you don't have bile. The liver makes 1 1/2 quarts of bile a day. Thus it needs a storage tank. That is the reason we have a gall bladder. If your gall bladder is removed, your liver cannot make bile fast enough to service a meal, so you will become fat depleted (fat around your hips and belly don't count). Without an ongoing source of good fat, you cannot keep your eyes in good repair. Thus if you don't have a gall bladder, you must take a bile supplement with each meal for the rest of your life.

Many are aware that vitamin A is important to vision. It is rare to find an internist/family practitioner or ophthalmologist that remembers that vitamin A is a fat-soluble vitamin. Without a gall bladder, you often become vitamin A deficient because without bile, you become deficient in the fat-soluble vitamins. Ophthalmologists and optometrist should be very interested in whether you have a gall bladder, but few ever ask.

Another important issues is nitric oxide. It is the master hormone of the body and also is responsible for dilation of blood vessels and bronchioles. If you don't have enough nitric oxide, your blood vessels can't dilate and you get high blood pressure. In addition, your lungs don't work efficiently so you don't move air in and out efficiently. This compromises your ability to have adequate oxygen.

Nitric oxide is made from an amino acid. You make amino acids by having your stomach acid break down the proteins you eat into amino acids. If you don't have enough stomach acid because you can't make it or because you are taking medications to keep you from making stomach acid, you can't break your proteins down into amino acids so you can't make nitric oxide. Thus you become unable to keep your vessels and bronchioles dilated. To make stomach acid requires iodine, zinc, and vitamin B1. Again we have the problem that doctors don't think about how they are contributing to glaucoma, brain fog, depression etc. when they prescribe pills to shut down your stomach acid. And certainly eye doctors aren't trained to consider that your stomach pills are the reason your glaucoma is out of control! No stomach acid leads to no amino acids and that leads to no nitric oxide and that means you can't dilate the vessels in your eye and retina.

Nor are doctors trained that the fluoride in your toothpaste is keeping you from making adequate stomach acid by inactivating the iodine you need to make stomach acid.

It should now be obvious to you that the nutrition necessary to make good neurons is critical to vision and the brain function. One must also have a functional circulatory system with oxygen from the lungs and glucose from the liver. The blood pressure must be high enough to put all of this uphill to the head.

If the pressure in the eye is high enough to compromise the circulation to the eye, it inhibits the arrival of vitamins, minerals, amino acids, fats, and oxygen necessary to the function of the retina and optic nerve as well as the parts of the brain that allow for vision to

work. This causes the neurons in the optic nerve to die.

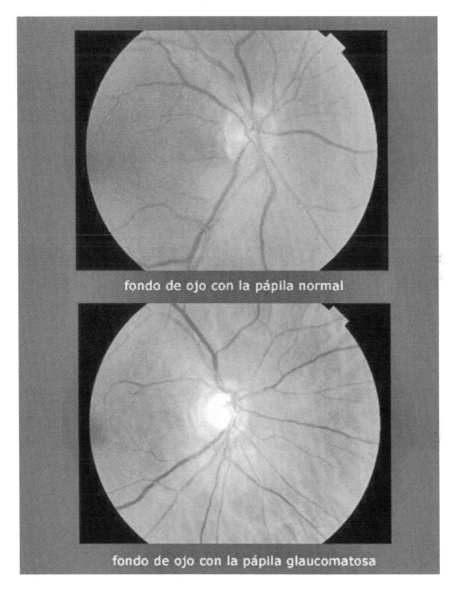

fondo de ojo con la pápila normal

fondo de ojo con la pápila glaucomatosa

Eventually this causes blindness. This is glaucoma.

The amino acid glutamate is the major signaling chemical in nature. All invertebrates (worms, insects, and the like) use glutamate for conveying messages from nerve to muscle. In mammals, glutamate is mainly present in the central nervous system, brain, and spinal cord, where it plays the role of a neuronal messenger, or neurotransmitter. In fact, almost all brain cells use glutamate to exchange messages. Moreover, glutamate can serve as a source of energy for the brain cells when their regular energy supplier, glucose, is lacking. However, when its levels rise too high in the spaces between cells—known as extracellular spaces—glutamate turns its coat to become a toxin that kills neurons.* http://www.dana.org/news/ cerebrum/detail.aspx?id=7376&p=3

When neurons become damaged, the glutamate is spilled out of the damaged neuron. This allows excess sodium, calcium and other things to enter the cell in large quantities. This causes an inflow of water. This makes the nerve cell die as its blood supply is compromised. This whole process is called a "**glutamate storm**".

One of the protective mechanisms against ongoing glutamate damage is vitamin B12 in large doses. What is considered "normal blood levels" of B12 may not be adequate in people with glaucoma. Having high blood levels of B12 is not damaging and thus you should not worry if blood tests find high levels of B12 while you are battling glaucoma.

Another protective mechanism occurs when you eat green apples or grapes. Apple juice is also useful. You should increase your intake of these fruits if you have glaucoma or other brain injuries.

Low Pressure Glaucoma

There is a condition where the pressure is in the "normal" range but the retina and optic nerve malfunction as if the pressure were high. This is called **"low-pressure glaucoma"** but is really a malfunction of the vascular/respiratory/liver/gall bladder/digestive system and really should be called **"optic nutritional deficiency syndrome"** or something similar to focus attention on where the problem really is.

What Causes the Pressure in the Eye to Increase?

In the opinion of this ophthalmologist, much of the teaching about glaucoma is incorrect because it ignores an understanding of the lymphatic system. To really understand glaucoma, you must understand the reason we have a lymphatic system and how it works.

The Cellular Sewage System (Lymphatics)

When cells place their garbage at the curb (push it into the extracellular space so it can be removed), most of it is moved into the venous capillaries. However, proteins are too large to fit there. Thus we have an entirely separate system to remove waste proteins.

Waste proteins can be considered cellular sewage!

The lymphatic system is dedicated to removing waste proteins. Thus it is our cells' sewage disposal system. These channels are tubes that connect the extracellular spaces around cells with a large vein (subclavian) that enters the heart just under the clavicles (collar bones). From here, it goes through the liver, into the bile, into the intestine and is removed from the body with your bowel movement.

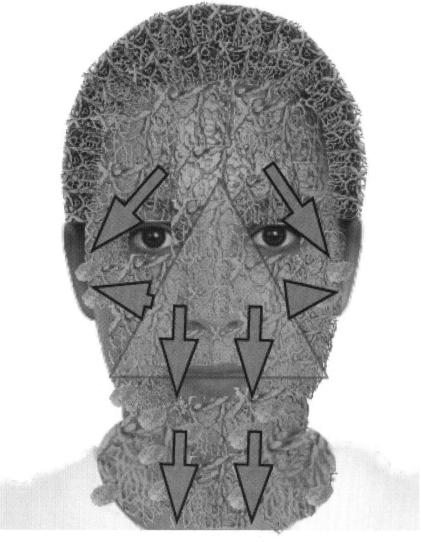

What is different about this system is that it has no heart or other pump to move the waste forward except in the head.

(In the head, the craniosacral pump assists in moving fluid in the lymphatics.) Instead, the tubes are surrounded by a circular muscle and by stretch receptors. When the tubes are stretched (such as by walking or moving your arms), they activate the circular muscles. This moves the sewage down the tubes much like squeezing a tube of toothpaste.

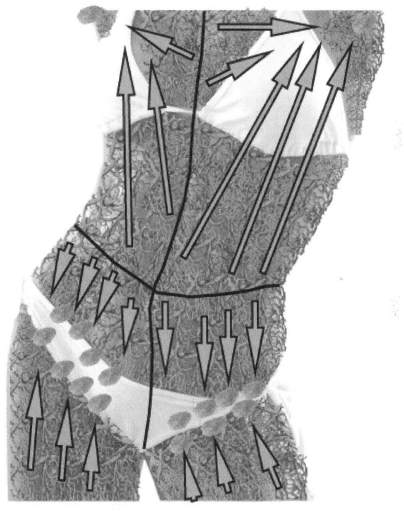

When you are inactive, the sewage isn't moved along the tubes. It can congeal in the tubes. Now your sewage system backs up just the way it can happen when your toilet gets stopped up by something too large to move through the sewer pipes. As the sewage backs up, it floods back into the extracellular spaces just as sewage floods your bathroom floor.

Can you see this in your mind? Your cells are surrounded by sewage. The sewage cannot be eliminated until you unstop the lymphatic tubes just as your toilet won't flush until you move the obstruction on down the pipes.

Sewage is a strong electron stealer. It significantly lowers the voltage in the extracellular space. This is reflected in a consistently low urine pH. That is because urine pH is a reflection of the voltage in your extracellular space. If it is consistently below 6.5, you likely have a stopped up lymphatic system.

People often notice that they are gaining weight or can't lose weight. This weight is often sewage instead of fat.

Another way to see if your sewage system is stopped up is to look at the clavicles (collar bones). They should be clearly visible. If you can't see your clavicles, you likely have lymphatic obstruction.

Allergies from Retained Sewage

Imagine what retained sewage does to you immune system. It drives it crazy! All of those damaged proteins are everywhere. It's like you fell into a pit of snakes and are struggling madly to get out. You strike out at anything that moves.

The longer that your lymphatics are obstructed, the more different antibodies you make until you become allergic to almost everything. Now you are called "chemically sensitive".

Surgery and Sewage

From any point on the body, the sewage must pass through a lymph node so that large particles and particularly bacteria can be filtered out before it reaches your blood stream as it flows into the subclavian vein just above your heart. Think of lymph nodes as sponges filled with antiseptics. You could also think of them as sewage treatment plants intended to clean up the sewage water before it comes back to your house.

What happens when a surgeon removes your lymph nodes? They take out some of the lymphatic pipes and their filters. Also scars interrupt the lymphatic sewer system and the acupuncture wires that bring voltage to the area. Now how is the sewage supposed to get cleaned and drained? It can't.

I Need a Plumber!

When you have allergies, you feel tired all the time, you are gaining weight and you can't see your clavicles, you likely need a plumber. Unfortunately, massage therapists can make it worse. Most of them are trained to work with muscles and not lymphatics. When you do deep massage on tissue filled with sewage, you often rupture the bulging lymphatic channels and the cells that are surrounded by sewage. What you need is a gentle method to contract the circular muscles that surround all lymphatic channels.

The ideal way to accomplish this is electronically. I use the Tennant Biomodulator with an attachment that has two balls on it. By gently following the normal flow of lymphatic sewage with the electrode, the tubes begin to move the sewage along. It is important to be sure the patient is hydrated. One must start where the system flows into the heart just behind the clavicles, Next open the neck channels. Then open the face and head channels. Now start down the body.

As you are opening the channels, it is important to be sure the lymph nodes are able to pass the fluid through them.

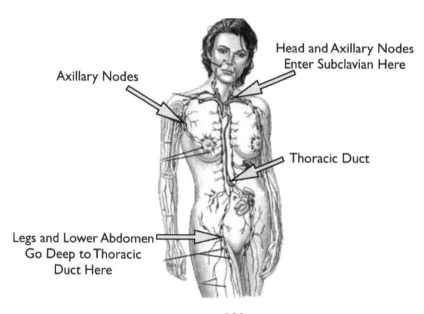

Head and Axillary Nodes
Enter Subclavian Here

Axillary Nodes

Thoracic Duct

Legs and Lower Abdomen
Go Deep to Thoracic
Duct Here

This can be accomplished by pressing on them like you are pressing the fluid out of a sponge.

The hardest one to open is the thoracic duct that takes the sewage from the inguinal area to the heart. It runs deep in the body next to the aorta. It requires some training to learn how to do this successfully.

Remember that the channels above the navel run to the nodes in the axilla (armpits) whereas the channels below the navel run to the inguinal region and then deep into the thoracic duct. When the thoracic duct is obstructed, people get fluid retention below the belly button. They think it is strange that they are getting fat just below the belly button and not above it. It's not fat; it's sewage.

The essential oil Bay Laurel is also helpful in getting the lymphatics to drain. So is a mini-trampoline.

The Eye is a Unique Part of the Lymphatic System

Remember that the reason we have a lymphatic system is to get rid of waste proteins because they are too large to fit into the venous capillaries. The waste proteins are from worn out proteins in the cells.

We replace the rods and cones in our retina every 48 hours, so we create a lot of "sewage" in our eyes. Therefore we need a special system capable of handling all this sewage. The inside of the eye is hollow so it has the room for all this sewage. To keep it flowing, some fluid is added by the lining of the focusing muscle (ciliary body) secreting what is known as "aqueous humor".   Thus aqueous humor is like extracellular fluid in the rest of the body.

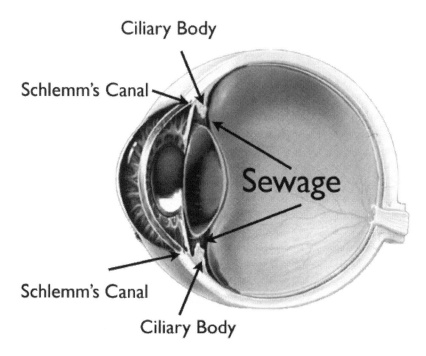

Remember that lymphatic tubes have large pores with flaps over them that allow the proteins to enter and be trapped inside the lymphatic tube. In the eye, this tube is in a circle around the front of the eye where the white sclera meets the clear cornea. It has a special name, "**Schlemm's Canal**". Here the sewage passes out of the eye into the general lymphatic system of the face as seen in the graphics on these pages. The sewage from the eyes flows from the corners of the eyes to lymph nodes in front of the ears. It then flows around the ear to a node behind the eyes known as the "water wheel". From here, it flows down channels along the sternocleidomastoid (strap) muscles of the neck to nodes just above the clavicles (collar bones). It then flows behind them into the final common port of the lymphatic system. This is where the lymphatics flow into a large vein (subclavian) and thus into the general circulation. It is then taken to the liver for detoxification and finally excreted by the

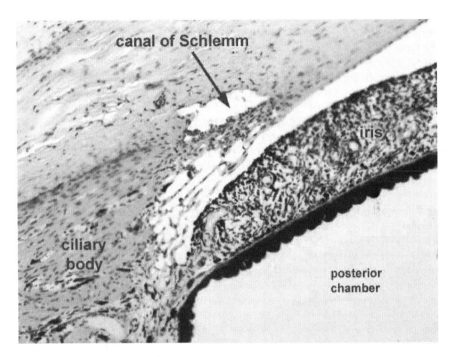

large intestine and kidneys.

The drainage system I have just described is similar to the one in your home. Consider a toilet upstairs in your home. Sewage is deposited in it. It then is flushed and goes down various sewage pipes until it finally exits your home and is sent to the sewage treatment plant (like your liver) where the proteins are broken down.

Now consider what happens when the sewer pipe that leaves you home is stopped up. When you flush the toilet, the water backs up, overflows and makes a mess on your bathroom floor. If you closed the bathroom door and it was water-tight and the toilet kept flushing, you would have "toilet glaucoma". The pressure of the sewage and water would keep building up inside the bathroom eventually causing destruction of the walls of the bathroom.   This is what happens to the nerves in your eyes when their lymphatic systems become obstructed. This is glaucoma.

If this were happening in your home, you would attempt to remove the obstruction in the sewer pipe between the bathroom and the street. That is what we should be doing with glaucoma.

Conventional Treatment of Glaucoma

Most conventional training in glaucoma ignores the lymphatic system and assumes that glaucoma is a malfunction of the venous capillary system. The conventional training in glaucoma is that the fluid manufactured by the ciliary body is intended to nourish the structures of the front of the eye since the cornea doesn't have blood vessels to bring it nourishment. As more nourishing fluid is made, it is intended to flow out of Schlemm's canal into the venous capillaries and thus maintain a normal pressure in the eye. Thus we are taught that Schlemm's canal is a part of the venous capillary system instead of a part of the lymphatic system.

When Schlemm's canal becomes obstructed for unknown reasons, pressure builds up in the eye causing damage to the nerves as they pass from the optic nerve to the retina. Treatment is then focused on decreasing the production of fluid from the ciliary body and/or increasing the outflow efficiency of Schlemm's canals. Drugs used to treat glaucoma are generally divided into those two groups: those that decrease fluid production and those that try to stretch Schlemm's canal so it will drain better. In general, those that are said to stretch Schlemm's canal are those that cause muscle contraction of the iris and ciliary body muscles. (They actually work by stimulating the circular muscles of the lymphatic channels.) They make the pupil very small. The muscle spasms induced by these drops can be very uncomfortable. The most famous of these drops are pilocarpine and carbachol. They are rarely used any more as drops that decrease fluid production are more abundant and profitable and cause fewer symptoms. However, these forgotten drops are a better in the sense that they encourage the drainage of the lymphatic channels where the real problem lies. Since their patents ran out years ago, it is hard for drug companies to make any money marketing them, so the newer drops have become standard of care.

An obvious problem with using drugs to decrease the fluid production in the eye is that the sewage gets thicker and more difficult to get into the lymphatic drainage channel called Schlemm' canal. Thus glaucoma treated in the standard way is characterized by a need to keep adding more and more medication to lower the pressure. All this does is increase the amount of sewage that can't get out of the eye. This retained sewage is an electron stealer so it lowers the voltage in the eye resulting in more rapid failure of the retina, lens, cornea, etc. with earlier onset of macular degeneration and cataracts.

Think of decreasing the amount of water you can have to flush your toilet. You decrease it by one pint (start the first eye drop). Then you decrease it by two pints (add the second eye drop). Then you keep decreasing it until you have no water left to flush the toilet. This is typical glaucoma therapy.

If the pressure cannot be lowered enough to stop damage to the nerve with the use of several eye drops (and occasionally oral medication as well), surgery is recommended. An effort is made to create a new channel where the fluid can flow outside the eye to lower the pressure.

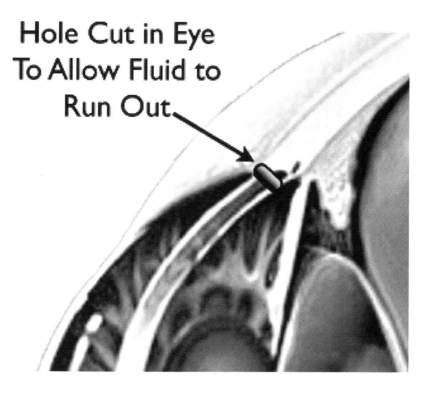

Hole Cut in Eye
To Allow Fluid to
Run Out.

Such surgical procedures have their own set of problems. If too much fluid flows out, the eye becomes too soft and cannot function. Scarring shut of the new channel is a constant problem and obviously makes the channel fail to lower pressure. Also, since there is an open tract from the outside to the inside of the eye, an infection inside the eye is a constant threat.

An ongoing effort over the last 30 years have been to create some sort of plastic valve that can be used to connect the inside and outside of the eye so fluid will flow out as necessary without having the valve/tube device scarring shut nor allowing too much fluid to flow out. As you might guess, there are significant mechanical problems with such devices including keeping them from migrating away from where you

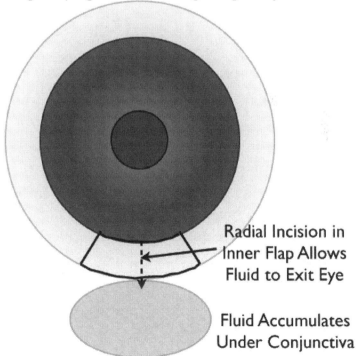

Radial Incision in Inner Flap Allows Fluid to Exit Eye

Fluid Accumulates Under Conjunctiva

put them.

Many years ago, I found a method to create such a channel that worked every time I used it and had no side effects. I discovered how to do it while removing cataracts in patients that also had glaucoma. I made the kind of two-stepped incision that I described in this book. I made it six mm. wide to accommodate the phakoemulsification (cataract removal) devices of that time. After removing the cataract and putting the lens implant in place, I took a diamond knife and split the inner layer of the two-stepped incision in a radial fashion. I extended this cut one mm. beyond the incision that was circumferential around the eye. Then I simply brushed the conjunctival flap over the area. No sutures were used. By constantly having the intraocular fluid flowing over the parted lips of the incision, it had no tendency to scar or heal. The tiny trickle of fluid under the conjunctival flap always controlled the eye pressure but did not cause any significant distortion of the conjunctival flap. There were no "thin blebs" as is often the case in similar filtration surgeries. There were no eyes that were too soft and no bleeding.

Patients loved not having to use eye drops after my surgery. They couldn't wait for me to fix the second eye. Then the government got involved. They decided that curing glaucoma while I was removing a cataract was "unnecessary surgery" and insisted I stop doing it. They made me give back all the money I had received for curing the glaucoma AND for removing the cataracts as well! My patients were furious, especially those that had the first eye cured and wanted the same in the second eye.

Since Medicare told me that curing glaucoma was unnecessary surgery, I created a form that the patients signed saying that if they wanted me to cure their glaucoma at the same time I removed their cataract, I would do so without any additional charge. However, the next time the Medicare "experts" reviewed my charts and found I was still doing the surgery at no charge, they told me if they caught me curing glaucoma again, I would be permanently banned from treating any Medicare patient. Thus I had to stop doing this wonderful procedure. "I'm from the government---I'm here to help you!" Yeah, right. The only people the government helped were those selling my patients expensive eye drops.

The Craniosacral Pump and Glaucoma

In the chapter on the Bowling Ball Syndrome, I discussed the craniosacral pump. This unique pump assists the lymphatic system in the skull. Thus it is critical in controlling eye pressures as well as helping remove fluid from your ears and brain.

I have seen eye pressures fall as much as 20 mm Hg (from 55 to 35 in open angle glaucoma) by just turning on the pump. Most people get a few mm, of improvement within an hour after correcting the Bowling Ball Syndrome to activate the pump.

The first thing that should be done in treating glaucoma is to turn the craniosacral pump back on. If you skipped it, go back and read the Bowling Ball Chapter.

A New Paradigm in Curing Glaucoma

What is meant by "curing" glaucoma. It is important that you realize that when the nerve fibers in the optic nerve die and your vision is significantly diminished, you will likely NOT get your vision back. If nerves are damaged, they can regenerate in some cases, but this can take 8-12 months. If they have become scar tissue, they cannot recover. Thus do not assume that following the steps I outline in this book will miraculously restore lost vision from glaucoma.

What is often possible is to stop the steady progress toward blindness and reduce or eliminate your need for eye medications to treat glaucoma. If you have the diagnosis of glaucoma and need to use daily medication to control it, you have glaucoma. If you had glaucoma but you can now go without drops or other treatments to control it, you are "cured". The analogy is diabetes. If your blood sugars are too high (over 135) and you lower them to 90 using diet and exercise, you are said to be "cured" from your diabetes. If your eye pressures are too high and causing damage and you use the things I am discussing in this book, you pressures may return to the levels where you no longer need medication. Like diabetes, you are said to be "cured" from your glaucoma. This does NOT necessarily mean that your vision returns to normal.

The things that are recommended to treat your glaucoma include:

1. Correct the Bowling Ball Syndrome and be sure your total body voltage is normal so the craniosacral pump will keep working.

2. Correct your total body voltage.

3. Correct lymphatic drainage from the head.

4. Correct your levels of humic and fulvic acids.

5. Correct your levels of stomach acid so you can make amino acids.

6. Correct your nitric oxide levels.

7. Eliminate any dental infections that are in the acupuncture circuits to the eyes to stop damage from thioethers and gliotoxins.

8. Be sure your blood pressure is high enough to get blood to the brain and eyes 120-140/80-90 unless you are diabetic or have kidney disease.

9. Be sure your liver is functional to provide glucose to the eyes.

10. Be sure your gall bladder works so it allows you to adsorb fats to repair your eyes. If you don't have a gall bladder, take bile with each meal.

11. Your eye doctor must follow you carefully to be sure there is no unrecognized damage occurring to the optic nerves.

12. Use only the amount of eye medication that is needed after the above are accomplished.

13. Don't stop or reduce your eye medication without being instructed to do so by your eye doctor.

12 Uveitis/Iritis (Ocular Inflammation)

The word uveitis is a compound of uvea and -itis. The term "-itis" means inflammation. The uvea is a layer of the eye that contains blood vessels. It is inside of the white sclera of the eye and outside of the retina. It comes from the Latin word "grape". If you remove the white sclera of the eye, the blood vessel coat looks like a grape. Thus uveitis is

Ciliary Body   Choroid (Blood Vessels)

Iris

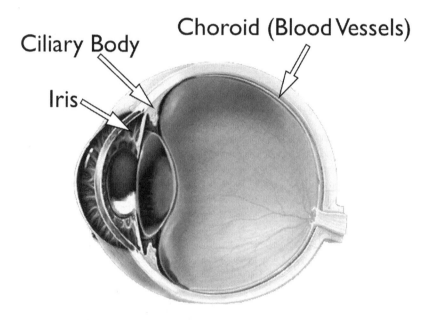

Uvea = Choroid + Ciliary Body + Iris

inflammation of the blood vessel coating of the eye.

The iris is the colored part of the eye that you see when you look at someone's eyes. Iritis means that the iris is inflamed.

Inflammation will always occur when you have an injury. For example, if you smash your finger with a hammer, the finger will swell, be warm, be painful, be red, and have a pulsing pain. Other types of injuries besides trauma are infections, chemical injuries, hemorrhage into tissue, and toxins.

Inflammation occurs primarily as a response to cell damage. When a cell is damaged, the body will move the voltage from -25 millivolts (operating voltage) to -50 millivolts (healing voltage). This is because it requires -50 millivolts to make new cells to replace the damaged ones. At -50 millivolts, the arterial capillaries dilate so they can dump the raw materials needed to make the new cells. These dilated arterial capillaries are what makes the tissue warm, swollen, red, and have a pulsing pain. After all the new cells are made to replace those damaged by the injury, everything goes back to normal.

However, what if there is ongoing injury? There will be ongoing healing with all the signs and symptoms mentioned above. A feature of this ongoing injury/healing pattern is that

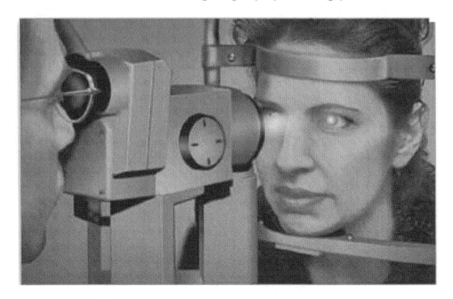

eventually you run out of voltage and thus can't make new cells to heal.

When the eye has experienced trauma, your doctors will be able to see the signs of the inflammation in the eye with the eye microscope (slit lamp). Note the gray collection of inflammation on the lens of the eye in the photo.

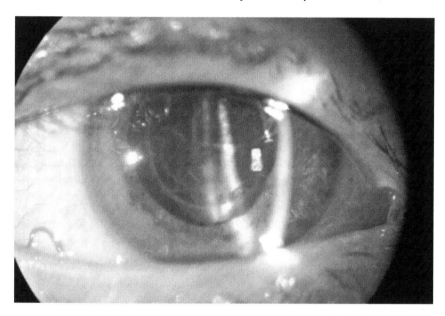

Doctors are taught to suppress this inflammation with steroid and other anti-inflammatory eye drops. It certainly makes the patient feel better, but it is not always a good idea to stop the body's efforts to heal itself.

However, if there has been no trauma, infection, hemorrhage, or chemical injury, there must be a toxin causing ongoing inflammation. Such ongoing inflammation leads to destruction of cells that cannot be repaired and thus loss of vision. This pattern of ongoing injury is characteristic of what are called autoimmune diseases.

Many years ago, doctors noted that sometimes tissues became inflamed and stayed that way. When such tissues were biopsied, they could see signs of cell destruction and inflammation. However cultures revealed no evidence of infections. Someone suggested that the body was attacking itself and thus was born the concept of autoimmune disease.

However there is another explanation for this scenario that I believe to be true. When voltage drops in cells, the amount of oxygen available to the cell drops. This is because the amount of oxygen that will dissolve in a cell is dictated by the voltage of the cell. As voltage drops, oxygen leaves the cell.

Each of us contains about a trillion micro-organisms. They are suppressed as long as oxygen is present. However, when oxygen drops, the "bugs" wake up. The first thing they want to do is to have lunch. And they want to have you for lunch. Since they don't have teeth to take a bite out of your cells, they put out digestive enzymes to dissolve the cells so they can get the nutrients from the cells. Of course this destroys the cells causing the usual inflammation we have been discussing.

The problem is that these digestive enzymes produced by the bugs are toxins to us. These toxins don't stay locally where they are produced. They enter our bloodstream and our acupuncture meridians. They go to distant places and cause the same cellular damage and inflammation they cause where they were produced.

A well-known example of this phenomenon is strep throat. When the strep bugs are having a picnic on our tonsils, the toxins they produce go to our heart and scar our heart valves. This is called "rheumatic heart disease". The same toxins can go to our knees and cause arthritis.

The same phenomenon can happen no matter where the bugs are having their picnic. Bugs in the gall bladder are known to cause damage to the brain. Bugs in the sinuses can cause arthritis. Bugs in the large intestine can do the same. However, the most common infections that cause so-called autoimmune diseases are in the teeth.

Each tooth is wired into an acupuncture meridian. You can find this chart in the dental chapter (Chapter 3). When you get a bacterial infection in a tooth, they produce toxins called thio-ethers. When the infections are fungal, the toxins are called glio-toxins. In addition, fungi produce particles almost indistinguishable from viruses called conidia. These are very destructive toxins (they have to be to dissolve a tooth). They pass along the associated acupuncture meridian causing

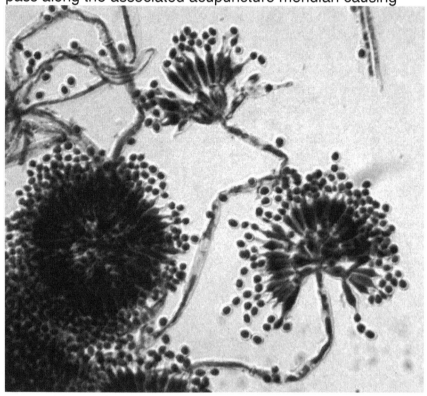

Conidia

damage to everything that is wired to that meridian.

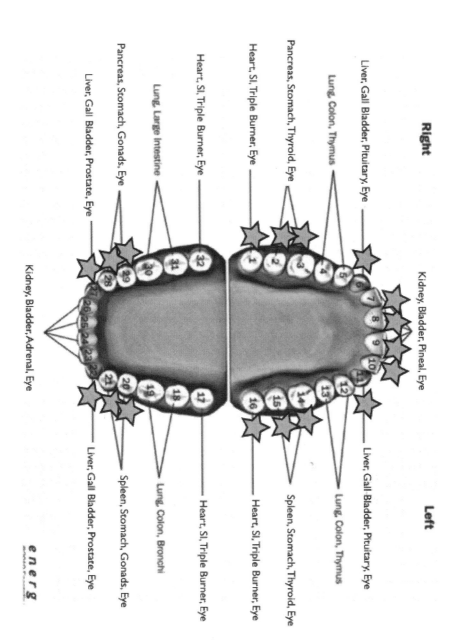

In the chart, I have put a star beside each tooth that is associated with the eyes. An infection in any of these teeth can cause uveitis. This is particularly true if you have a root canal in one of these teeth.

In traditional Chinese medicine, the acupuncture wires that provide voltage to the eyes are Triple Burner, Liver, and Bladder. I have also found that the Spleen Meridian is the one most commonly involved with macular disease, particularly when the macula has a pre-retinal membrane (called cellophane maculopathy).

Chronic uveitis of the eye can usually be resolved by removing the infection from the teeth that are in the meridians mentioned above. Remember that root canal teeth are ALWAYS infected and are the most common offender in causing so-called autoimmune diseases.

In the image, you can see the teeth that are on the acupuncture wires that deliver voltage to the eyes. When these teeth are infected, they carry toxins and/or conidia to the eyes. These toxins or fungal particles damage cells in the eyes. This stimulates the typical healing reaction of going to -50 millivolts and dilation of the arterial capillaries. There is also a pulsing pain. In the eye, there is also a sensitivity to light.

Because there is an ongoing infection in the tooth/teeth, there will be an ongoing reaction in the eye(s). Usually the affected eye is on the same side as the infected tooth. Then you get the diagnosis of chronic uveitis.

In traditional medicine, you will be treated with steroids in the form of eye drops. In more severe cases, you will be put on oral steroids or even chemotherapy drugs to stop your immune system from reacting to the toxins.

Of course all you really need to do is get rid of the chronic infection in the teeth, liver, bladder, or spleen. Once you stop the production of the toxin, your uveitis is gone! Usually a trip to a knowledgeable dentist is all you need to do to cure your uveitis.

13 Summary

This book is about healing eye diseases. It builds on the series of Healing is Voltage, The Textbook and Healing is Voltage, The Handbook. Both are available from www.tennantinstitute.com.

Although modern medicine is sometimes almost miraculous with acute problems, the results of treating chronic diseases are disappointing. The World Health Organization rates medical outcomes in the US as 37th in the world. It isn't affordable and it doesn't work well. It has left us with many diseases that are considered untreatable.

A different paradigm considers that we get well by making new cells. Making new cells requires -50 millivolts of power and all the raw materials needed to make a cell that works. In addition, one must get rid of toxins that damage new cells as they are made. Approaching illness as an inability to make new cells that work correctly is a paradigm that allows us to heal things that are usually considered untreatable.

One of the great things about this method is that there are no side effects. Giving the body good nutrition, correcting digestion so you can absorb these nutrients, and providing the body the voltage it is missing allows you to make good cells. For example, there are no side effects to correcting your stomach so it can turn proteins into the amino acids that you need to make cells.

These principles apply to eyes as well as the rest of the body. If we begin treating eye diseases before the damage turns into scar tissue, we can reverse cataracts, macular degeneration and glaucoma. Uveitis is treatable by eliminating hidden sources of infections, usually hiding in the teeth.

Contact Details:

Jerry Tennant, MD, MD(H), MD(P)
Tennant Institute
9901 Valley Ranch Parkway E.
Suite 1015
Irving, TX 75063
972-580-1156 phone
972-580-0715 fax
www.tennantinstitute.com
info@tennantinstitute.com

BioModulator Distributor:

Senergy Medical Group
9901 Valley Ranch Parkway E.
Suite 1019
Irving, TX 75063
972-580-0545 phone
www.senergy.us
biomodulator@senergy.us

Abdomen BioTerminal   75, 101,109
Absolute Risks   153
Acidic   10, 11, 23
Acidic Alkaline   10
Acupuncture   33, 46, 55-60, 63, 64, 71-74, 83, 85, 88
Acupuncture System   33, 46, 55, 56, 58-60, 64, 71, 85
ADHD   163
ADP   15, 44, 45
Advanced AMD   201
Aflatoxin   165, 166, 169
Age-Related Eye Disease   200
Age-related Macular Degeneration   199-201
Alcoholic   24. 167
Alkaline   10, 20, 39
Allergies   227, 228
ANA   17
Anaerobic   8
Analog Perineural Nervous System   46, 50, 55
Anti-prostaglandin Drugs   181
Antibiotics   162, 163, 167-170
Appendicitis   54
AREDS   200
Arginine   152
ARMD   199
Arsenic   28
Ascomycete   166
Aspergillus   165-167
Assess Mode   60, 88, 92
Asthma   53, 163
Asthma Insomnia   151
ATP   15, 16, 44, 45, 88, 99
Automatic Infinity   91, 92, 96
Autonomic Nervous System   147, 149
Avastin   202
Ayers, Margaret   147
Base BioTerminal   9, 60, 61, 76, 77
Battery   90
Bay Laurel   230

Beauchamp   164, 165
Beauchamp, Antoine   164, 165
Becker, Robert   46-51, 207
Becker, Rollin   135, 136
Bernard, Claude   164, 165
Betaine   158, 198
Bevacizumab   202
BIA   43
Binkhorst, Cornelius   176
Bio Cranial Therapy   139, 142, 145
Biological Impedance Analysis   43
Biologically Closed Electric Circuits 59
BioModulator   55, 60, 71, 77, 78, 88, 197, 211, 213
BioModulator Distributor 249
BioTerminal System   70
BioTerminals   65-67, 69, 87, 88, 92, 96, 98, 101, 106, 109
Bipolar   204, 206, 208
Birth   195
Bladder   42, 43, 53, 54, 64, 73-77, 84, 86, 93, 102, 107
Bladder Tesla   102, 107
Blood   8, 9, 13, 17-19, 37, 50-53, 56, 59, 88, 92, 97, 99,
106, 151, 154
Board Of Homeopathic And Alternative Medicine MD   1
Bone   136, 137, 139, 142, 143, 145
Bowling Ball Syndrome   133, 139, 142, 147-149, 238, 239
Boyd, Robert   139, 142, 143
BRAIN   16, 34-36, 42, 50-52, 60, 71, 86
Brain BioTerminal   86
Brain Waves   146
Bronchitis   53
Bryan, Nathan S.   154
Burmeister, Mary   63
Bursitis   52
Cancer   12, 17, 37, 38, 47, 163-167, 170, 171
Candida   162, 165, 168
Canola   36-42, 105
Capacitance   204
Capacitors   25, 32, 44, 31-34, 72,73, 74, 79, 204
Capacitors Yin Coils Yang   73

iii

Cataracts	191, 194-197
Catchfly Plant	166, 167
Cells	8, 10-16, 18, 19, 24, 25, 34-37, 42-44, 48, 50, 51, 56, 88, 92, 99, 105, 203, 206-208, 211-213
Cellular Sewage System	224
Chakra	60, 61, 64, 65
Chest	53, 65, 66, 68, 69, 75
Cholesterol Obesity	151
Choyce Mark VIII	178
Choyce, Peter	177-180, 182
Christy, Norvell	173
Chronic Fatigue	163
Circuits	31-33, 59, 63, 71-73, 77, 86-88
Clostridium	103
CNS	134
Coils	32, 73
Cones	199, 200, 203-205
Conidia	169, 245, 247
Connective Tissue Planes	57, 58
Copeland	176
Corboy Award	2
Cranial	133-137, 139, 140, 142, 143, 146
Cranial Bone Movement	136
Cranial Osteopathy	134
Craniosacral Pump	135, 137, 139, 141, 146, 226, 238, 239
Craniosacral Therapy	136
Crown BioTerminal	76, 77, 86
CSF	134
Curing Glaucoma	237-239
Diabetes	163, 194
Diodes	29, 30, 56
DNA	157, 166, 167, 198
Dropped Nucleus	188
Dry Macular Degeneration	200, 202
Duke-Elder, Stewart	177
Edison, Thomas	71
Electrons	9, 11, 14, 15, 19-25, 27-30, 32-34, 44-46, 51, 55, 56, 58, 59, 70, 71, 77, 85, 87
Enderlein, Gunther	164

Endothelial	156
Ergonom	17
Excimer Laser Surgery	183
Exercise	23, 77
Eye Chakra	61, 64
Eye Surgery	173, 174, 181
Fascia	56, 58, 64, 67, 71
Fat	25, 32, 34-37, 42-44, 88, 104-106
FDA Statement	89
Fermentation	160, 164, 168
Fibrous	45, 46, 50, 51, 55, 56, 58
Five Element Theory	83
Fluoride	99
Free Radical Antioxidant	10
Fulvic Acid	159-161, 171
Fungus	159-161, 163-169, 171
Fyodorov, Svyatoslav Nikolayevich 183, 184	
Galin, Miles	173
Gall Bladder	42, 43, 53, 64, 73, 74, 76, 77, 84, 86
GERD	163
Glaucoma	194, 215, 221-224, 233-235, 237-239
Glucose	8, 15, 36, 42
Hays, Doug	142
Headache	52
Heart	16, 37-39, 47, 53, 61, 71, 73-75, 84, 85, 93, 94, 219, 225, 228-230
Heart Chakra	61
Hellman, Monte	173
Howell, Dean	142
HT Chest BioTerminal	66
Humic	159-161, 171
Hypertension	163
Impedance	204
Infinity	91, 92, 146
Inflammation	241-244
Intermediate AMD	201
Intraocular Lenses	175-177, 179, 181
IOL	175, 177
IOL Surgery	175

Ionic Transfer Of Electrons   59
Iritis   241
Jin Shin   62, 64, 67
Kabbalah   70
Kidney   54, 74, 75, 84, 85
King Method   63
King, Glenn   63
Koch, Robert   163
Krebs   15
L-arginine   152, 156, 157
L-forms   18, 99, 104
Lactic Acid   8
Langevin, Helene M.   57
Large Intestine   16, 54, 58, 73, 75, 84, 86
Laryngitis   52
LASEK   185
Laser-Assisted Sub-Epithelial Keratectomy   185
Leukemia   163, 165, 170
Liquid Crystals   26, 27, 34
Little Wings   144, 145
Liver   35-37, 39, 41-43, 51, 53, 73, 74, 76, 77, 84-86, 94, 102, 106, 107, 247
Livingston-Wheeler, Virginia   164, 165
Low Pressure Glaucoma   224
Lucentis   201, 202
Lung   37, 38, 58, 73, 75, 84-86
Luo Points   65, 73, 77
Lyme Disease   19
Lymphatic System   224, 227, 230-233, 238
Lymphoma   163, 170
Macular Degeneration   106, 107, 109, 151, 158, 199-202, 208, 209, 211-214
Macular Photocoagulation Study   201
McDonald, Marguerite   185
McIntyre, David   173
Microprocessor   30, 31, 34, 44
Migraine   141, 163
Moorfields Hospital   177
Morgan, Thomas Hunt   48

Murai, Master Jiro   61, 63, 64
Mycobacterium   163
N-type   29, 30
Neuro-Cranial Restructuring   142
Nitric Oxide   150-152, 154, 156-158, 220, 221, 240
NO Index   154
Non-Hodgkin Lymphoma   170
Nördenstrom, Björn   50, 59, 207
Obesity   42, 53
Olbrich, Kurt   165
Order of Saint Sylvester   2
Order of Santiago   4
Order of St. Gregory   2
Osteopathic Medicine   133, 135
Oxygen   8, 9, 15-17, 45, 88
P-type   29, 30
Pain   8, 13, 15, 52-54, 73, 88
Parallel Tuned Circuits   32, 72
Pasteur, Louis   164, 165
Pearce   182
Penicillin   163, 168-170
Pericardium   53, 73, 74, 86, 106
Peripheral Cytoskeleton   31-34
Perspex   182
Phase Angle   43
Phase Contrast Microscope   18, 19
Photo-refractive Keratectomy 185
Photoreceptors   203-206, 208
Phytoplankton   213
Plastic Fats   35, 36, 42
Pope Benedict XVI   3
Precision Cosmet   179, 182, 183
Probiotics   168
Prostate Specific Antigen (PSA)   166
Rapeseed   36-39
Raw Materials   172, 198
Rayner Optical   177, 179, 182
Regeneration   46, 47, 51, 196

Relative Risks	153
Resonating Circuit	31, 34, 72
Retained Sewage	227, 234
Revenko, Alexander	144
Ridley, Harold	177, 182
Rife, Royal	162
Rods	199, 203-205
Russian SCENAR	208, 211
Sanjiao	73, 74
SCENAR	144, 145, 208, 211
Schiotz	215-218
Schlemm	231, 233, 234
Schumann	139
Schwann	50
Sciatica	54
Semiconductors	27, 28, 30, 56
Senergy Medical Group	249
Sewage	224, 226-234
Simoncini, Tullio	165
Small Intestine	54, 73-75, 84
Soy	99, 104, 105
Spitfire	182
Spleen	37, 53, 73-75, 84, 85
Spores	160, 162, 164, 166, 167, 169
Srinivasan	184, 185
Statin	194
Still, Andrew Taylor	133, 135
Stomach	53, 68, 73-75, 84, 101, 106, 109, 212
Strampelli	182
Sutherland, W. G.	135
Ten-8	91, 92
Tennant	55, 60, 71, 77, 78, 88, 212
Tennant BioModulator	55, 60, 71, 77, 78, 88, 89, 145, 146, 149, 229
Tennant BioTerminals	88
Tennant Institute	4, 249
Tesla	31, 33, 34, 71-73, 77, 86, 88, 97, 101, 102, 104, 106, 109, 204
Tesla Circuit	71, 77, 86, 88
Tesla Resonating Circuits	73

Tesla, Nikola   31, 71, 72
TKM   63
TMJ   140
Tonopen   217, 218
Trans Fats   35, 38, 42
Transistors   30, 31, 56
Trauma   195
Treatment of Age-Related Macular Degeneration   201
Trokel, Steven   185
Ultraviolet Light Damage   180
Upledger, John   136
Uveitis   195, 241, 246, 247, 248
Vedas   60
Verteporfin   201
VISX   4
Vitamin B1   152, 158
Vitamin B12   152
Vitamin B2   152
Vitamin B3   152
Vitamin B5   152
Vitamin B6   152
Vitamin B7   152
Vitamin C   152
Vitamin C   194
Vitamin E   194
Vitamin K1   152
Vitamin K2.   152
Vitamins   160, 161, 167
Voltage   5, 7, 8-17, 19, 21-23, 27, 30, 33, 34, 36, 44, 48,
51, 55, 59, 60, 64, 68, 71, 77, 87, 88, 92-95, 97-107, 109, 160, 161, 164, 167,
168, 171
Warburg, Otto   164
Wet Macular Degeneration   200-202
World Health Organization   248
Zand, Janet   154
Zinc   104, 105

Made in the USA
Lexington, KY
24 May 2018